The Aging Network
Programs and Services

Sixth Edition

About the Author

DONALD E. GELFAND, PHD, is Professor Emeritus at Wayne State University. His interests span both basic and applied areas of aging. He is coeditor of the recent volume *End of Life Stories: Crossing Disciplinary Boundaries* (Springer, 2005) and author of *Aging and Ethnicity: Knowledge and Services* (Springer, 2003). Dr. Gelfand has conducted research on major programs and service delivery areas in aging and attitudes and use of services by many ethnic populations. His current activities focus on end-of-life issues. He has served as Coordinator of the Wayne State University End-of-Life Interdisciplinary Project, which has developed courses and research on this important topic and has published research on the attitudes of Latinos toward end-of-life services.

The Aging Network
Programs and Services
Sixth Edition

Donald E. Gelfand, PhD

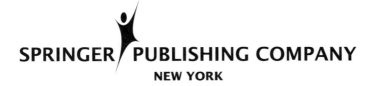

SPRINGER PUBLISHING COMPANY

NEW YORK

Springer Publishing Company, Inc.
11 West 42nd Street
New York, NY 10036

Acquisitions Editor: Helvi Gold
Production Editor: Sara Yoo
Cover design by Joanne Honigman
Typeset by Daily Information Processing, Churchville, PA

06 07 08 09 10 / 5 4 3 2 1

Library of Congress Cataloging-in-Publication Data

Gelfand, Donald E.
  The aging network : programs and services / Donald E.
Gelfand —- 6th ed.
    p. ; cm.
  Includes bibliographical references and index.
  ISBN 0-8261-0206-9
  1. Older people—Services for—United States.
  [DNLM: 1. Old Age Assistance—United States. 2. Health
Services for the Aged—United States. 3. Social Planning—United
States. WT 30 G316a 2006] I. Title.

HV1461.G44 2006
362.60973—dc22

2005031310

Printed in the United States of America by Bang Printing.

Contents

Preface to the Sixth Edition

Textbooks for Social Problems courses in Sociology departments usually include a chapter on "An Aging Society." Rather than seeing the increased numbers of older persons in industrialized society as a social problem, we can regard this change as a wonderful achievement. The fact that the majority of individuals in countries such as the United States now live past the age of 65 is worth celebrating.

Although we celebrate this increased longevity, there is no denying, however, that it does bring new demands to bear on society. These include how to provide programs and services for older people with cognitive, physical, and social needs. These needs must be met in a manner that ensures the continued viability of government and private agencies, but does not place extraordinary demands on family members or the older persons themselves.

The programs and services discussed in this book have primarily been put in place since the 1960s. Although no fundamental change in the configuration of aging services in the United States took place during the 1990s, the National Family Caregiver added to the Older Americans Act (OAA) in 2000 recognized the need to support families involved in extensive caregiving for older relatives.

It can be expected that the Older Americans Act will continue to be reauthorized without controversy in the foreseeable future. However, as the competition for budget priorities at state and federal levels indicates, the services for older people will not receive large increases during the first part of the 21st century. Specific attention will instead be focused on "problems" such as Alzheimer's disease or the high cost of prescription drugs. Services such as senior centers and adult day care will have to be resourceful to meet their needs. There may be also be increasing pressure to shift the costs of some programs and services to older people and their families. Programs outside the OAA such as Medicare and Social Security

will be the subjects of increased efforts to control their costs for beneficiaries and taxpayers.

As in previous editions, this volume provides information on regulations of such programs as Medicare and Medicaid, but no effort is made
to cover every aspect of every program and service. My intent is to high-
light the primary components of specific programs and services and to
emphasize the most recent and important changes. Although positive or
negative aspects of existing programs and services are mentioned, a comprehensive evaluation of all income maintenance, health, and aging network programs is beyond the scope of this volume.

The last authorization of the Older Americans Act forms the basis of
most of the discussion. Many of the publications available from the organizations listed in the Appendix provide additional details about programs at the federal, state, and local levels.

I have oriented the writing of this book to a number of audiences.
The first group is students who are interested in working with older populations. Making choices about jobs and careers requires an understanding of what programs and services now exist, the opportunities they
provide for an individual, and their past and future directions. The second group is individuals who are working with older populations in the
many varied settings described in the chapters. For these staff members,
a basic knowledge of the programs and services now available and how
they relate to each other can improve their ability to help older individuals, who often require assistance from a number of programs and services.
This understanding is also important in any effort to expand programs
and services. Finally, based on previous editions, I have learned that many
individuals find the chapters helpful in their decisions about utilizing specific programs and services for themselves, and/or family members.

I am grateful to the staff of Springer Publishing Company, especially
Ursula Springer, for their continued support in the development of this
volume. I am particularly grateful to my wife, Katharine, for her patience
during the process of preparing this edition.

Introduction

The number and complexity of programs and services for older people continue to grow, as does the population they aim to serve. Television, radio stations, and movies aim their products at an 18–49-year-old age group, but the increasing wealth in the hands of older people and baby boomers is becoming more and more evident. As another sign of change, The American Association of Retired Persons altered its name to AARP, as many older people continue to work long past conventionally defined ages of retirement. On the other hand, many individuals now have the means to retire early and to live with the resources available to them.

There is thus a "market" for "senior services" delivered by both public and private entities. The potential of this market is evident in the fact that the 2006 Medicare prescription drug coverage will be administered by private insurers and not by the federal Medicare agency. The number of products that are sold through AARP has also increased and has caused some to question the purpose of this huge organization.

The diversity of programs and services for older persons is probably a positive development as long as consumers can understand what is being offered to them and at what cost. Throughout this book, I try to clarify the goals, target populations, and important components of specific programs and services. Each chapter also outlines the background, past and present funding, and some of the interesting variations in these programs and services as they are delivered to older populations across the country.

ORGANIZATION OF THE BOOK

Part I focuses on the present status of older Americans and the general thrust of programs and services in aging. After a brief glimpse at the characteristics of older adults in Chapter 1, Chapter 2 moves into an extensive examination of federal legislation authorizing programs and services for the aged. The major emphasis is on the provisions of the Older Americans Act.

In Part II, the complex but crucial topic of income maintenance and health insurance is explored, including both the burgeoning private pension plans and major public programs such as Social Security, Supplemental Security Income, Medicare, and Medicaid.

Part III provides details on major programs in aging, ranging from information and referral efforts to crime prevention programs throughout the United States.

Part IV moves on to a discussion of the enlarging service delivery systems for the elderly, including senior centers, the growing in-home services, and adult day care centers. This part concludes with an examination of the always controversial and increasingly varied types of long-term residences now available for seniors.

Having discussed the myriad efforts that fall under each of these headings, Chapter 16 provides a brief opportunity to reflect on the factors that have allowed for such rapid development of these programs and services and their probable future.

PART I

The American Elderly and Programs

Older Americans are increasingly diverse in ethnic backgrounds, religion, income, and education. Chapter 1 presents relevant statistical data on the older population as an important background to the planning and development of programs.

With this groundwork laid, Chapter 2 plunges into an in-depth examination of the programs and services for the aged. The focus is on the programs authorized and funded through the Older Americans Act and on related programs stemming from a variety of federal and state legislation. The complexity of existing legislation will be quickly evident, but an understanding of titles and acts discussed is imperative for students and practitioners interested in the field of aging.

CHAPTER ONE

The Older American

THE ELDERLY POPULATION

Before we examine any programs, some attention must be paid to the number and characteristics of older Americans. This foundation should enable the reader to assess critically the specific programs and services discussed in the remaining chapters of this book. Rather than viewing characteristics statically, the focus will be on the changing status of the elderly during the 20th century.

Size of the Population

If "older persons" are defined as individuals over the age of 65, this group represented 12.4% of the U.S. population in 2000. As large as this population is (35 million people), the proportion of older persons in the United States decreased slightly between 1990 and 2000. The majority of older individuals (53%) were between the ages of 65 and 74 and an additional 35% were between the ages of 75 and 84. Although the population over the age of 85 represented only 12% of the older population and 1.5% of the total American population, this group experienced the most rapid growth during the 1990s. During this decade, the population over the age of 85 increased by 38% compared to a growth rate of only .2% among individuals aged 65–74. This differential reflected the decisions many couples made during the Great Depression of the 1930s not to have children during that disastrous economic period. Even with the slowed growth in the proportion of the older population, older individuals are still expected to account for 20% of the American population by 2020 as the "baby boomers" enter their later years beginning in 2011 (U.S. Census Bureau, 2001).

Life expectancy for individuals born in 2003 reached an all time high of 77.3 years. White men born in 2003 could expect to live 75.4 years on average and White women 80.5 years. Although the gap in life expectancy between women and men has declined since the 1979 peak of 7.8 years, the greater life expectancy of women than men is expected to last into the 21st century. These life expectancy figures hide some important intergroup differences. Minority elderly still have lower life expectancy rates than White elderly: Black males born in 2003 have a life expectancy 6.2 years shorter than White males born that year, and Black females have a 4.7 year shorter life expectancy than their White counterparts (National Center for Health Statistics, 2005).

Perhaps more important than life expectancy at birth is the life expectancy of individuals who reach the ages of 65 and 85. An individual who reached 65 in 2002 had an average life expectancy of an additional 18.2 years: 19.5 years for females and 16.6 years for males (Administration on Aging, 2005.) At age 85, the average life expectancy for men was 5.2 years and for women 6.8 years (Administration on Aging, 2003).

There were already 12 million persons over the age of 75 in the mid-1980s. The over-85 population will increase from approximately 3.6 million in 1995 to 6.1 million in 2010 and 9.6 million by 2030. The result of this increase is that the population over the age of 85 will have grown from 1.4% of the population in 1995 to 5% of the population in 2050 (Federal Agency Forum on Aging Related Statistics, 2004).

The proportion of African American and Latino elderly in the American population will continue to grow during the 21st century. As a result of the "aging" of each of these groups, their median age will continue to rise. In 2003, the median age for Whites was 37.3 years, Blacks, 30.6 years; American Indian/Alaskan Natives, 28.9 years; Asians, 33.7 years; and Latinos, 26.7 years (U.S. Census Bureau, 2003). By 2030, it is expected that more than one-quarter of older Americans will be from minority backgrounds (Administration on Aging, 2005).

In 2003, 12.5% of the White population in the United States was over the age of 65. Among other racial and ethnic populations there were smaller proportions of older people: 8.1% among the Black population, 6.2% among Native Americans and Alaskan Natives, 8.3% among Asians, 5.5% among Native Hawaiians and Pacific Islanders, and 5.2% among Latinos (U.S. Census Bureau, 2003).

Health Status

The major problems of older persons are not acute illnesses, but chronic conditions that affect their functioning. Problems in functioning are usually assessed on the basis of the relative inability of the individual to carry out basic Activities of Daily Living (ADLs: bathing, dressing, feeding oneself, reaching and using the toilet, and transferring between bed and chair). The Instrumental Activities of Daily Living (IADLs) include the ability to perform household tasks such as meal preparation, housecleaning, money management, shopping, getting around in the community, and using the telephone. The proportion of older persons who cannot perform the ADLs is not increasing. In 1996 Siegel projected that the number of disabled older persons would triple by 2040 (Siegel, 1996). The commonness of disability is illustrated by the fact that in 1997, over half of the older American population reported having at least one physical or nonphysical disability (Administration on Aging, 2005).

Chronic conditions are the cause of a large proportion of problems in functioning among older persons. Among the most common chronic conditions are arthritis (32/100 persons), hypertension (49%), heart disease (31%), sinusitis (15.1%), and diabetes (15%) (Administration on Aging, 2003). Beyond the pain associated with a condition such as arthritis, the impact on older persons may include difficulty in feeding themselves, cooking, taking medicines, or even walking. The other conditions listed above can also have a major impact on the daily lives and activities of older people. As the American population continues to age, the prevalence of other diseases may dramatically increase.

LIVING PATTERNS

There are now 1.5 million nursing home beds in the United States, but the over-65 population in nursing homes still represents less than 5% of the total number of older American adults. One of the most striking statistics of recent years is the increasing proportion of older individuals who are maintaining their own households. The percentage of older persons living alone, however, varies by age. Most significantly, about half of women over the age of 75 were living alone in 2003 (Federal Interagency Forum on Aging Related Statistics, 2004). About 30.8% (10.5 million) of all noninstitutionalized older persons in 2003 lived alone (7.8 million women, 2.7 million men). They represented 39.7% of older women and 18.8% of older men.

There are also variations by race and ethnicity in the proportions of older persons who live alone. Overall, non-Hispanic White and Black women were most likely to be living alone in 2003. The number of elderly living alone also reflects the dispersal of families over a wide area. Poorer families consistently live closer to their elderly relatives. It has also been shown that family income is positively related to the use of long-term care residences for elderly parents. Poorer families who cannot afford nursing home care are thus more likely to have an older family member living with them.

Rural states, such as Iowa, Arkansas, and Missouri, continue to have high proportions of elderly. In these states, younger families have moved to more urbanized regions and have not been replaced by any significant numbers of new residents. Although a proportion of the elderly have joined in the migration to the suburbs, many suburban residents have grown old in their neighborhoods. As a result of the "aging in place" phenomenon, half of the elderly were living in the suburbs in 2002 as compared to one-third in 1960. Almost one-quarter (23%) of older persons lived in non-metropolitan areas (Administration on Aging, 2003). As research continues to show, older people tend to remain in communities where they have lived for a long period of time. Compared with 48% of younger individuals, only 23% of older persons moved between 1995 and 2002.

Cultural Backgrounds

Although many senior advocacy groups speak out against stereotyping, there is a continued tendency to discuss the elderly as a homogeneous group whose values and beliefs are defined by their age. In reality, the cultural backgrounds among the present generation of individuals over 60 are enormously varied. The U.S. census counted 30 million individuals who were born outside the United States. Two demographic facts about this population are important for the field of aging: (1) the median age of foreign-born individuals is above 52 and (2) the foreign-born population is very diverse. It includes substantial numbers of Latinos from Central and South America; Asians from Korea, China, Cambodia, India, Laos, and Vietnam; and Haitians and Caribbean Islanders (Gelfand, 2003). Differences in cultural attitudes toward aging and utilization of services, as well as a lack of fluency in English among foreign-born elderly, may create problems for providers attempting to implement aging programs.

Education

The minimal educational background of many present-day elderly also creates problems for service providers, who must understand that many of them have limited verbal, writing, and reading skills. Programs that involve extensive reading and discussion may thus not be practical for many elderly. At a more basic level, many elderly will have difficulty understanding and following instructions on medication and may utilize their medication improperly. As the differentials in educational background between the elderly and the general population become less distinct, these problems will abate. The improvement in educational background is already evident if data for the period from 1970 to 2003 are examined. During this period the percentage of persons over the age of 65 who had completed high school rose from 28% to 72%. There are still substantial differences in the educational backgrounds of White and minority elderly. Among older Whites, 74% had graduated from high school in 1994, whereas only 52% of African American elderly and 36% of Latinos had high school diplomas (Federal Interagency Forum on Aging Related Statistics, 2004).

Employment and Income

Recent changes in American work patterns have not been of major benefit to many American and foreign-born elderly. The inability of these older adults to obtain higher education during the early 1900s relegated them to careers as blue-collar workers. Men and women whose work has centered around low-paying jobs have meager financial resources for their old age. Low wages have meant low Social Security benefits and inadequate or nonexistent pensions. Part-time and intermittent work has prevented many women from accumulating enough "quarters" to qualify for Social Security.

Many of the elderly being served by present-day programs have limited ability to pay for costly services. Income maintenance programs such as Supplemental Security Income (SSI), Medicare, food stamps, and housing subsidies have helped to raise the income floor of the elderly. In 2003, only 10.2% of individuals over age 65 fell below the federal poverty level, but this figure does not adequately convey the income problems faced by minority elderly. Although less than 10% of White elderly (8.8%) had less than poverty level income in 2003, the comparable figures were 23.7% among Blacks, 14.3% among Asians, and 19.5% among Latinos. In 2005, the federal poverty level was only $9,570 for one person and $12,830 for two persons. For 38% of Black retirees and 40% of Latino retirees, Social Security is their only source of income. In contrast, only 18% of White retirees depend entirely on Social Security for all of their income (Andrews, 2005).

Although their status has improved on many fronts, the elderly still suffer from a variety of deficits that require the assistance of formal and informal interventions. After examining the existing programs and services, I will return in Chapter 16 to a discussion of the challenges faced by the aging network attempting to provide these programs and services.

REFERENCES

Administration on Aging. (2003). *A profile of older Americans: 2003*. Retrieved November 15, 2004, from http://www.aoa.gov

Administration on Aging. (2005). *A profile of older Americans: 2004.* Retrieved June 6, 2005, from http://www.aoa.gov

Andrews, E. (2005, March 20, 21). G.O.P. courts Blacks and Hispanics on Social Security. *New York Times,* A15.

Federal Interagency Forum on Aging Related Statistics. (2004). *Older Americans 2004: Key indicators of well-being.* Hyattsville, MD: National Center for Health Statistics.

Gelfand, D. (2003). *Aging and ethnicity* (2nd ed.). New York: Springer Publishing Co.

National Center for Health Statistics. (2005). *2005 fact sheet—life expectancy hits record high.* Retrieved March 1, 2005, from http://www.cdc.gov/nchs/pressroom/05facts/lifeexpectancy.htm

Siegel, J. (1996). *Aging in the 21st century.* Washington, DC: National Aging Information Center.

U.S. Census Bureau. (2001). *The 65 years and over population: 2000.* Washington, DC: Author.

U.S. Census Bureau. (2003). *Selected age groups for the population by race and Hispanic origin for the U.S.: July 1, 2003.* Retrieved November 23, 2004, from http://www.census.gov/Press-Reslease/www/releases/img/eb04-98-table2.xls

CHAPTER TWO

Legislative Bases for Programs and Services

The present generation of elderly benefits from the "categorical" programs, designed to serve all individuals who fall into a specifically defined group (in this case older adults) and from generic programs that benefit all age groups. This chapter will review the legislation underlying existing aging programs. Besides highlighting the important legislation, it will examine other sources of programs and services for the aged and the major funding mechanisms underlying these services. Attention will focus on the legislative initiatives and programs formulated at the federal level and implemented by state and local governmental units.

The major influence on programs for older adults has been the Older Americans Act (OAA) initially passed by Congress in 1965. Many of the features of the Act were influenced by the 1961 White House Conference on Aging. The Act has been amended 11 times; the 12th amending was signed into law by President Clinton in 2000 and reauthorized the OAA through the end of fiscal 2005. The 2000 amendments maintained the seven basic titles of the Act but consolidated some of these titles and included a few new initiatives.

A major change that needs to be highlighted was the incorporation of cost sharing provision into the Act. Until the 2000 amendments the Older Americans Act had one unique element: it was not means-tested (income). All individuals over the age of 60 were eligible to use its programs and services. As already noted, there has always been the question of whether this open-ended attitude toward OAA services was ethically correct or financially prudent. As the population of older people grows dramatically, the basic question of how to pay for services will increasingly be asked. It is already being asked in regard to health care but financial support for OAA programs will also become more of an issue during the next 50 years.

During the late 1980s, there was sentiment on the part of many provider agencies for initiation of cost-sharing on the part of clients, based on their incomes. The agencies asserted that cost-sharing would increase their income and allow them to expand more programs and services. Other groups argued that cost-sharing would stigmatize OAA programs and reduce the participation of many elderly, particularly minority elderly (Gelfand & Bechill, 1991). The 1992 amendments had an increased specificity on the need of state and local providers to target their efforts toward the most "needy" older individuals, including needy minority elderly.

Cost-sharing was finally authorized in the 2000 Older Americans Act amendments. Agencies are now allowed to charge for some of their services based on the recipients' income. No assets such as value of their homes or savings are counted. Older individuals can self-declare their income and agencies cannot ask them to fill out any forms or provide any documentation as verification. Agencies are also required to develop a plan to ensure that cost-sharing does not discourage any older persons from obtaining the services they need. This problem could result from a feeling of stigmatization on the part of older individuals who now view services they receive as an indication that they are not able to provide for themselves financially. Other individuals may also hesitate to ask for agency help because they do not want to declare their income.

In 2000, cost-sharing was not allowed for a variety of programs and services. These included information and assistance, outreach, benefits counseling, case management, elder abuse legal assistance, consumer protection, and congregate and home-delivered meals. The full impact of the new cost-sharing provisions will always be difficult to determine, but they are clearly a major change from the non-means tested approach of the 1965 OAA. Pennsylvania's OPTIONS program, which provides long-term care services, is an example of cost-sharing. The costs borne by the care recipient are based on the person's income and the cost of the services being delivered. Older persons whose income is below 125% of the federal poverty level are exempt from cost-sharing (Pennylvania Department of Aging, n.d.).

The appropriateness of cost-sharing may become clearer through the examination of each of the specific programs and services of the OAA. In this chapter, the individual Titles of the Act will be described. Important differences between the 2000 OAA and previous versions will be delineated. The specifics of individual programs and services are provided in subsequent chapters.

THE OLDER AMERICANS ACT

Purpose of the Act

The basic purpose of the Older Americans Act is to "help older persons" by providing funds to the states for services, training, and research. All three of these activities are to be coordinated through the Administration on Aging (AoA). As part of a reorganization plan, the Office of Human Development Services was abolished in 1991. The Administration on Aging was a major component of this Office. As a result of the reorganization, the AoA became an independent agency that reports directly to the Secretary of the Department of Health and Human Services.

TITLE I: OBJECTIVES

In 1965, the goals of the OAA were couched in sweeping language that encompassed 10 difficult but laudable objectives:

1. An adequate income
2. The best possible physical and mental health
3. Suitable housing
4. Full restorative services
5. Opportunity for employment without age discrimination
6. Retirement in health, honor, and dignity
7. Pursuit of meaningful dignity
8. Efficient community services when needed
9. Immediate benefit from proven research knowledge
10. Freedom, independence, and the free exercise of individual initiative (Butler, 1975, p. 329).

In 1978, a new stress was placed on the provision of community services that enabled the older person to make a choice among a variety of subsidized living arrangements. In 1987, objective 7 was altered to emphasize the participation of older persons in "meaningful activities" and objective 10 was expanded to guarantee "protection against abuse, neglect and exploitation." The 1992 amendments expanded objective 4 not only to include impaired elderly, but also to support services for the caregivers of impaired elderly.

The target population of the OAA was originally individuals over the age of 65. In 1973, without extensive opposition in Congress, this was changed to the age of 60. Part of the logic in the reduction of the eligible age was that the programs and services developed under the Act's provisions would assist older individuals in pre-retirement planning. A review of the Act's history and titles reveals that the Administration on Aging has become responsible for the operation of an extensive service delivery program for older people (Gelfand & Bechill, 1991).

TITLE II:
ADMINISTRATION ON AGING

A direct outcome of the enactment of the OAA was the organization of the Administration on Aging (AoA). Directed by the Assistant Secretary of Aging, AoA is charged with carrying out the provisions of the OAA. The Assistant Secretary is appointed by the President and confirmed by the U.S. Senate.

As can be seen by even a quick perusal of the OAA, the responsibilities of the AoA are extensive. They range from providing information on problems of the aging to planning, gathering statistics, setting policies, and coordinating ongoing efforts in aging at federal and local levels with private and public organizations. The data-gathering responsibilities of the AoA were increased by the 1987 OAA amendments. These responsibilities include gathering information on services funded, individuals served, and the extensiveness of support by the Area Agencies on Aging for elderly with the greatest economic and social needs, particularly low-income minority elderly, low-income elderly in general, and frail older persons. This latter group would include individuals with mental as well as physical handicaps.

The 1978 OAA amendments outlined a role for the AoA as an advocate of aging programs throughout the federal government (Sec. 202a). Sections 202 and 203 also stressed the importance of the Assistant Secretary's intervention in a variety of planning, regulatory, and coordinating activities.

Recent reauthorizations of the OAA stress the Assistant Secretary's role and responsibility to consult with other federal agencies concerned with programs that have an impact on the elderly. The 1992 amendments established an Office of Long-Term Care Ombudsman Programs within the Administration on Aging. The mandate of this office is to recommend policies regarding ombudsman programs. One staff person is also to be designated by the Assistant Secretary as a Nutrition Officer responsible for the administration of all nutrition programs funded through the OAA. In addition, the Act authorized the establishment of a National Center on Elder Abuse and a National Aging Information Center.

TITLE III:
GRANTS FOR STATE AND
COMMUNITY PROGRAMS IN AGING

Title III is the most important component of the Older Americans Act. This title outlines the types of services that should be provided at the local level in order to develop "comprehensive and coordinated services" enabling older adults to maintain "maximum independence" (Sec. 301). The basic foundation for providing these services is an agency designated by the governor of each state with responsibility for aging services. In many states, this agency has been a newly form Office on Aging. State offices on aging are not always provided mandate to oversee all aging programs; some remain within a' tablished departments. In 28 states, the Office on Aging is man services department, whereas in another 21 stat Aging is independent.

The agency designated by the governor is respo. opment of a 3-year statewide plan for serving the el service areas must be designated by the agency, and local A Aging (AAAs) must be established. Within each of these a agency has latitude in outlining geographic service areas. In n. these areas have coincided with health and mental health plann.

The AAA develops its own 3-year service plan, which must L mitted for approval by the state agency. An area agency can be a un. county, city, or town government or even a private nonprofit agenc. Preference must be given to an already established Office on Aging. In 2000, 655 AAAs were in existence across the country. In 13 states, the state agency is also the AAA.

Since its original passage, the categories of services that need to be addressed in an AAA service plan have grown. The 1987 amendments added disorders related to Alzheimer's disease, and the 1992 amendments added case management as an appropriate service. The State and AAA plan must set "specific objectives" [306a(5)(A)(I)] to identify a variety of older individuals who need services:

- rural elderly
- older individuals with greatest economic need
- older individuals with greatest social need, with a particular emphasis on low-income minority elderly
- severely disabled elderly
- elderly whose ability in English is limited
- older persons suffering from Alzheimer's and related disorders

The area plan must demonstrate coordination of services provided through the AAA and services provided through other agencies, including community action agencies.

In the 1975 amendments, four priority areas were noted: transportation, in-home services, legal services, and home repair and renovation programs. In 1978, the three priority areas were access services (transportation, outreach, information, and referral), "in-home services" (homemakers, home health aides, visiting, and telephone reassurance efforts), and legal services. In 1987, the OAA required that the area plan demonstrate coordination of in-home, access, and legal services with ongoing activities of other community organizations working with Alzheimer's disease patients and their families. In 1992, case management was classified as an access service.

Supportive Services

Supportive services as defined in the Act include a wide range of programs, ranging from health care efforts to transportation, housing assistance, residential repairs, and an ombudsman program designed to "investigate and resolve complaints by older individuals who are residents of long-term care facilities" (Sec. 307). The 1981 amendments also authorized a number of new initiatives, including efforts formerly undertaken by other federal agencies. These efforts include crime-prevention and victim-assistance programs, the installation of security devices, job counseling programs, and the Senior Opportunities and Services Program (formerly operated by the Community Services Administration), which focused attention on the poor elderly.

The 1992 amendments added a number of supportive services to the already substantial list. These included:

- translation services for non-English speaking elderly
- representation in guardianship cases
- counseling for older individuals who provide care to adult children
- expanded types of therapies
- expanded counseling in regard to various types of insurance, "lifestyle changes, relocation, legal matters, leisure time, and other appropriate matters"
- support services for family members caring for older individuals needing long-term care
- services for individuals who are currently, or may become, guardians
- services that will "encourage and facilitate interaction between school-age children and older individuals . . ." [Sec. 313].

In the 2000 amendments, in-home services for frail elderly and assistance for special needs of older persons were classified as supportive services. If the need for funds is less for supportive services than for nutrition, states could transfer 30% of supportive service funds to nutrition programs.

In 1981, the Senate introduced an amendment to the OAA requiring specific state programs for geographically concentrated groups of non–English-speaking elderly. A full-time AAA employee was to be assigned to provide counseling, as well as information and referral, to non–English-speaking older persons. This staff member would also have the responsibility of ensuring that local service providers are "aware of cultural sensitivities and . . . take into account effectively linguistic and cultural differences" [Sec. 307(a)(20)].

Nutrition Programs

Until 1978, nutrition programs comprised Title VII of the Older Americans Act. In 1978, Title VII was deleted and reclassified as Section C of Title III. Whereas in 1978 the Act stressed the provision of congregate meals, the 1981 amendments asked for increased flexibility only, noting that primary consideration be given to congregate meals settings but allowing an AAA to award a grant to an organization that provided only home-delivered meals. Another major change was the restriction by Congress on the diversion of funds earmarked for nutrition to supportive services such as recreation, information, and assistance or counseling. The ability to use funds for supportive services that was part of the 1978 amendments was important in allowing nutrition programs to expand their efforts. Congregate programs accept donations, and home-delivered meals programs are permitted to charge for their services based on income levels in the community. The funds obtained by these charges can be used for supportive services and to facilitate access of the older person to the meal sites. The 1992 amendments included a new initiative to offer school-based meals for older persons who volunteer in schools, and fund intergenerational, social, and recreational programs for older volunteers [Sec. 316]. OAA funds can be used to pay 85% of the costs of these meals or for intergenerational activities that involve older people and students. Under the 1992 OAA amendments, 30% of the nutrition funds could be transferred between congregate and home-delivered meals. This amount was raised to 40% in the 2000 amendments.

Senior Centers

In 1981, Title V, dealing with multipurpose senior centers (first included in the 1973 amendments), also became part of Title III. The 1981 amendments again recognize that the multipurpose senior center is not a separate service entity, but rather a "community facility" for organizing and providing the gamut of social and nutritional services authorized by the OAA. In 1978, the House-Senate conferees were unwilling to authorize separate funding for multipurpose senior centers. This unwillingness represents the viewpoint that centers are part of the social services delivery network of the state and its AAAs (U.S. House of Representatives, 1978). In fact, Title III stresses that "where feasible, a focal point for comprehensive service delivery" should be created with "special consideration" given to "designating multipurpose senior centers as such focal point" [Sec. 306(a)(3)]. The AoA is authorized to make grants to the states for construction, acquisition, and renovation of buildings usable as senior centers. The federal government can insure mortgages for these centers, and social services funds can be used for the centers' operating costs.

The 2000 amendments also continued the emphasis of the 1992 amendments on disease-prevention and health-promotion services. The 1992 amendments included an extensive list of 12 disease-prevention and health-promotion services that range from health assessments and screening through nutritional counseling, physical fitness and dance, music, and art therapy.

The major innovation in the 2000 amendments was the introduction of the National Family Caregiver Support Program as a major component of Title III. This program consolidates some of the earlier elements of Title III mentioned above into a concerted effort to provide information and assistance to family members who are caregivers for older people as well as grandparents who are caring for young children. For the first year of the program $125 million was authorized and the funds could be used to provide information about available services, as well as counseling and training for caregivers. The states were expected to allot these funds on the basis of an intrastate formula that gave priority to the number of people over age 70 in an area. Each state was also expected to provide a match of 25% for the funds they received and other federal funds could not be used for this match.

Although the exact amount of funds expended for each of these Title III activities will vary from state to state, the 1987 amendments required that the state plans specify a minimum percentage of funds that each AAA must spend on each service and program. In addition, documentation is now required from AAAs on how service providers will meet the needs of low-income minority aged. In this effort, service providers must attempt to provide services to low-income minority elderly in proportion to their representation in the population of older adults in the area. Thus, if low-income minority elderly are 10% of the elderly population in an area, 10% of the services providers' funds should be targeted to their needs.

TITLE IV:
TRAINING, RESEARCH, DISCRETIONARY PROJECTS, AND PROGRAMS

Title IV has been a mainstay of training and research efforts in the field of aging. This includes efforts of state and local governments as well as a variety of public and private organizations. Under Title IV-A, diverse training projects have been funded, including short-term training courses, in-service institutes, and seminars and conferences. Concern about a shortage of trained personnel to serve the aging has grown, and the 2000 amendments emphasize funding of training for workers in a variety of fields including mental health and services for the blind.

TITLE V:
COMMUNITY SERVICE EMPLOYMENT

Title V of the 1981 OAA was formerly Title IX, originally added to the OAA in 1973. The stress in Title V is on coordination of projects underway in a variety of state, federal, and private agencies. The title also attempts to delineate the role of groups that contract to provide community service employment for older adults. As in the past, the priority recipients of community employment services are individuals over 55 who are unemployed or whose prospects for employment are limited. Individuals with an income equal to or less than the intermediate budget for retired couples developed by the Bureau of Labor Statistics are eligible for Title V programs. The OAA also stresses second-career training in "growth industries and in jobs reflecting new technological skills" [Sec. 502(e)(2)].

TITLE VI:
GRANTS FOR NATIVE AMERICANS

This title authorizes funds for Native American tribes to develop social and nutritional services for the aged if Title III programs are not already providing adequate services. The enactment of a separate title on Indian elderly represents an enlargement of the 1975 amendments to the OAA, which encourage states to directly fund Indian tribes interested in providing services to the elderly if these services are not already available. In 1987, OAA amendments explicitly recognized the needs of older Alaskan natives and Native Hawaiians as well as programs and services needed by older Native Americans. The amendments also strengthened the role of native tribal organizations in the provision of services and provided guidelines for application for and use of Title VI funds (Sec. 614). A similar section (Sec. 623) relates to funding for Native Hawaiians.

TITLE VII:
VULNERABLE ELDER RIGHTS
PROTECTION ACTIVITIES

This new Title VII was adopted in 1992, but some of its components were formerly included in Title III. Title VII has four major components: The "State Long-Term Care Ombudsman Program" [Sec. 712]; "Programs for Prevention of Elder Abuse, Neglect and Exploitation" [Sec. 721] "State Elder Rights and Legal Assistance Development" [Sec. 731]; and "State Outreach, Counseling and Assistance Program for Insurance and Public Benefits" [Sec. 741]. These sections reflect concern that older people do not receive the benefits to which they are entitled, as is certainly the case with the Supplemental Security Income program. The title thus aims to "expand State responsibility for the development, coordination, and management of statewide programs and services directed toward ensuring that older individuals have access to, and assistance in securing and maintaining, benefits and rights" (Congressional Record, 1992, p. 8989). In the effort to assist AAAs and other state agencies in understanding issues related to the rights of older people, the state has to appoint a focal point for state-level policy review, analysis, and advocacy on these issues. Personnel who will be involved with these issues must be designated, including a "State legal assistance developer." The State Outreach, Counseling and Assistance Program helps older individuals compare available Medicare supplemental policies and obtain those benefits to which they are entitled. The program will also help older people compare life insurance, other insurance, and pension plans. When needed, the program will help the individual obtain benefits and refer the older client to legal assistance when appropriate.

FUNDING OF AGING PROGRAMS

Prior to 1973, funding for aging programs and services was minimal. Gold (1974) has characterized the programs and services supported in the 1960s as community demonstrations. The passage of the Nutrition Services Act in 1972 was thus a major breakthrough in its focus on large-scale direct services for the elderly. Until 1981, Congressional appropriations for activities under the OAA had increased dramatically, enabling the implementation of a wide range of programs and services.

During the 1980s, federal funds appropriated for Title III-B programs increased by only 10%. In FY 1990, Congress appropriated only 74% of the funding it authorized (Kutza, 1991). Although funding is at a much higher level than it was in the 1980s, it still remains inadequate to meet the needs of provider agencies. In 2005, $354 million was appropriated for supportive services of Title III, $387 million for congregate meals, and $182 million for home-delivered meals (Administration on Aging, n.d). This funding gap has forced states and localities to increase their financial support for many programs and services authorized through the Older Americans Act.

Geographic Funds

A crucial element in the development of aging programs and services is the formula used by individual states to distribute funds they receive from the federal government. The percentages of minority elderly, poor elderly, and individuals over age 75 have all been common elements in intrastate formulas. As a U.S. General Accounting Office study (1990) noted, the Administration on Aging did not officially approve or disapprove particular state formulas, and there was a large diversity of formulas. These formulas came under scrutiny when a Florida court ruled that the state's formula was discriminatory. The 1992 OAA amendments required that intrastate formulas be developed in consultation with Area Agencies on Aging and in accordance with guidelines set by the AoA Assistant Secretary. AoA must also approve all intrastate formulas.

The formulas must take into account the distribution of older people in the state as well as the geographic distribution of older persons with "the greatest economic need and older individuals with greatest social need, with particular attention to low-income minority old individuals" [Sec. 305(a)(2)]. Each state must specify how it will meet the needs of low-income minority elderly in each local area.

"Economic" and "social" need were more precisely defined in the 1992 amendments than they had been in earlier OAA authorizations. "Economic need" was defined as an income below the federal poverty line. "Social need" can be caused by a variety of factors that include (a) physical and mental disabilities, (b) language barriers, and (c) cultural, social, or geographical isolation, including isolation caused by racial or ethnic status that (i) restricts the ability of an individual to perform normal daily tasks or (ii) threatens the capacity of the individual to live independently [Sec. 102]. Local Area Agencies on Aging must indicate the extent to which they have been able to serve older persons who fit these criteria.

Block Grants

Funds to support programs for the elderly are available through many federal agencies besides the Department of Health and Human Services. Large proportions of these funds are not specifically targeted for elderly groups but allow the elderly to be considered as an eligible population.

Decisions on allocation of these funds increasingly are made at the local level. This is characteristic of General Revenue Sharing, Community Development, and the new block grants enacted in fiscal 1982. As opposed to categorical grants, block grants distribute funds directly to the state. States are allowed to utilize these funds for specific broad areas, but with little federal regulation and reporting. Among the initial block grants enacted in FY 1982 were the Alcohol/Drug Abuse and Mental Health block grant, the Social Services block grant, the Energy Assistance block grant, and the Community Services block grant. These contained funds that could be used to support programs for older persons. The Reagan administration expressed a strong interest in including other programs within the block grant framework.

In 1981–1982, federal regulations for block grants specified only that a public hearing be held concerning the allocation of block grant funds, and that a report be sent to the federal government explaining how the block grant funds would be targeted on the basis of need. No specific evaluation on the effectiveness of distributed funds was planned. In specific programs, some strings were attached to the block grants by Congress. In the Alcohol/Drug Abuse and Mental Health block grant, states were expected in FY 1982 to continue to fund mental health centers at a "reasonable" level, and the funds could not be shifted among the three programs of this block grant until 1982. The block grants thus offered the states and local communities increased flexibility to determine program and population priorities: that is, whether the elderly are a group requiring special attention and funding.

The Social Services block grant is a replacement for Title XX of the Social Security Act. In 1974, Title XX was included in the Social Service Amendments to the Social Security Act, replacing Titles IVA and VI. Title XX funds were distributed according to the size of the state's population. The state was required to design a package of services and define the eligible population. Among the services for the aging that received funding in various states under Title XX were adult day care, foster care, homemaker services, nutrition programs, senior centers, protective services, services in long-term care residences, and funds for comprehensive community mental health centers.

Despite the seeming comprehensiveness of this list, the number of programs and services for the elderly funded under Title XX was limited.

This limitation resulted from federal requirements that states fund at least a specific group of "mandated services" and a ceiling that Congress placed on Title XX allocation.

Federal mandated services included adoption, day care for children, early periodic screening, diagnosis and treatment of chronic and potential illnesses, employment counseling, family planning, foster care for children, information and referral, protective services for abused and neglected spouses and children, and services to the disabled, elderly, and blind. These required services were deleted from the block grant, but there is still a strong feeling in many states that Title XX was originally designed to provide services to children because of its origins in Titles IVA and VI of the Social Security Act.

Title XX had five goals:

1. To help people become or remain economically self-supporting
2. To help people become or remain self-sufficient
3. To protect children and adults who cannot protect themselves
4. To prevent and reduce inappropriate institutionalization
5. To arrange for appropriate placement and services in an institution when this is in an individual's best interest (State of Maryland, 1978).

In order to avoid rancor in distribution of block grant funds, many states have chosen to maintain these goals. Funds to help older people pay home energy bills are available through the Low Income Energy Assistance Program. Individuals are eligible if their income does not exceed 150% of the federal poverty level of 60% of the median income of the state.

From an overall perspective, the additional services in Title III and Title IV demonstrations of the OAA reflect the burgeoning number of issues currently under discussion in the field of aging, particularly caregiving issues, legal rights, and elder abuse. One important change is the perceived need not only to provide services to older people, but also to the individuals who assist them. The increased specificity about greatest needs, and the requirement that the Assistant Secretary of Aging approve the intrastate funding formula, indicate a concern that programs and services are not equitable in their distribution. The implementation of the Older Americans Act, through a variety of existing and new programs and services, is what is now termed the "aging network." The structure of this informal network (Figure 2.1) includes federal, state, and local organizations that provide important programs and services for older people.

National Aging Services Network

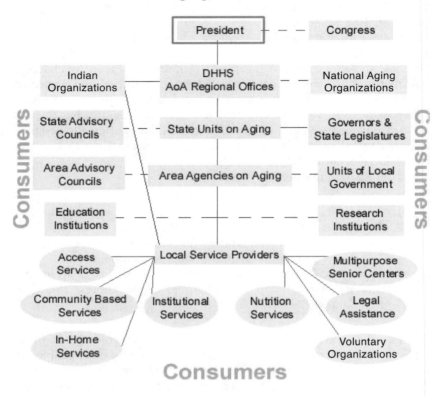

FIGURE 2.1 National Aging Network.
Source: http://www.aoa.gov/prof/agingnet/leadership/leadership.asp

REFERENCES

Administration on Aging. (n.d.). *FY 2006 budget request.* Retrieved February 9, 2005, from http://www.aoa/gov/about/legbudg/current_budg/legbudg_current_budg.asp

Butler, R. (1975). *Why survive: Being old in America.* New York: Harper & Row.

Congressional Record. (1992). H.R.2967, 102 Congress, 2nd session, 138 Congressional Record, No. 130, Part II.

Gelfand, D., & Bechill, W. (1991). Older Americans Act: A 25 year review of legislative changes. *Generations, 15,* 19–22.

Gold, B. (1974). The role of the federal government in the provision of social services to older persons. In F. Eisele (Ed.), Political consequences of aging. *Annals, 415,* 55–69.

Kutza, E. (1991). The Older Americans Act of 2000: What should it be? *Generations, 15,* 65–68.

Pennsylvania Department of Aging. (n.d.). *OPTIONS program: Community based long-term care.* Retrieved June 8, 2005, from http://www.aging.state.pa.us/aging/cwp/view.asp?a=284&Q=173869&agingNavDLTEST=%7C4364%7C4421%7C

State of Maryland, Department of Human Resources. (1978). *Proposed FY 1979 Title XX Comprehensive Annual Services Plan.* Annapolis, MD: Author.

United States General Accounting Office. (1990). *Older Americans Act: Administration on Aging does not approve intrastate funding formulas.* Washington, DC: U.S. Government Printing Office.

United States House of Representatives. (1978). *Conference report No. 95–1618: Comprehensive Older Americans Act Amendments of 1978.* Washington, DC: U.S. Government Printing Office.

PART II

Income Maintenance Programs

The system of income maintenance in the United States is a complex, fragmented one. Responsibility is divided among all the units of government and the private sector. The system, if it can be called one, was created step by step over a period of many years. Programs were created or modified, and occasionally abandoned, as circumstances arose or changed. A prime example of incrementalism, the system is an illustration of block-by-block building to meet recognized need, often without careful consideration of the impact of the new developments upon existing programs.

The present system of income maintenance is characterized by program distinctions made on the basis of:

- *Governmental responsibility:* Some programs are federally operated, others are operated by the states, and some are operated privately.
- *Financing:* Appropriations from the general revenues of government, both federal and state, finance some programs. Others are financed out of reserve funds created by insurance premiums.
- *Relationship to the workforce:* Some programs are limited to those who have an attachment to the workforce, whereas others are available without such connection.
- *Eligibility:* There are some universal programs with no means test. Others are limited to those who pass a means test, with the test varying from program to program.
- *Participant contribution:* Some income maintenance programs are financed in part from contributions or taxes imposed upon the individual. Others are financed by payments made by the employer or from governmental tax revenues.

The interplay of these factors not only creates confusion in grasping what the system includes, but also reveals the weaknesses in the system. There is some duplication of coverage, and there are also gaps and omissions. There are serious variations in the level of adequacy of payments among the programs. Although some elements in the overall system are well financed, others are less secure. A number of programs operate in obscurity, thus limiting their utilization by many potential clients.

Elements in the U.S. income maintenance system will be reviewed here from the point of view of the resources available to help older people. The programs will be considered in terms of governmental response to the risks to which people are exposed, which include:

- Growing old without adequate income
- Being unemployed and without income
- Being ill and unable to work in order to support oneself and one's dependents
- Being ill and unable to pay for medical care

Chapter 3 will focus on the risks of inadequate income for the elderly. The role of income maintenance programs in periods of illness and existing medical care coverage programs will be the focus of Chapter 4.

CHAPTER THREE

Age, Employment, and Income Maintenance

GROWING OLD WITHOUT ADEQUATE INCOME

The risk of becoming old and being unable to work is one of the most serious situations that people face. Although many elders retire from employment voluntarily, the tendency is for people to remain employed for as long as possible. Older workers who become unemployed because of obsolete skills, or because companies go out of business or consolidate, very often do not find other jobs. These workers are thus less able to plan their entry into retirement than are those who have been steadily employed.

Historically, the aged have been recognized as in need of help, as evidenced very early by the enactment of poor laws. In the 1920s, the impact of the rigorous poor law was eased by the introduction of the Old-Age Pension, a means-tested program of aid usually available at age 70. These programs were liberalized and incorporated into the Social Security Act (SSA) of 1935 in the form of grants to the states for old-age assistance. The SSA also established the Old-Age Benefit Program. Because it was apparent that it would be several years before that program would actually provide benefits, the means-tested program was the major source of income for the elderly.

Progressive liberalization in the retirement provisions of the Social Security Act has resulted in that being a primary source of income for many older persons since 1951. The old-age assistance program gradually diminished in size, to the point that it provided assistance for only a small proportion of the aged. In 1974, the old-age assistance program was federalized and merged with similar programs for the blind and disabled as part of the Supplemental Security Income (SSI) program.

Before these programs are examined in greater depth, it is important to view them in relationship to each other. The old-age benefit program under the Social Security Act is generally considered the basic program. Not only is it broad in its coverage, but the rights that are accumulated under the program are "portable," that is, the rights are cumulative throughout one's lifetime and are carried from one employer to another. Social Security has become the cornerstone of protection in old age. Although benefits have increased in adequacy, the amount provided inevitably falls short of what many people will need or want in their retirement years. It is at this point that the private pension system enters the picture.

The government has acted to encourage the growth of private pensions with a view toward provision of income in addition to Social Security benefits. Social Security was never intended to provide benefits that were measurable against a specific standard of adequacy. The adequacy of Social Security income is obviously improved when combined with private pensions. Employers are now encouraged to establish private pension programs. Workers are given an opportunity to negotiate with employers in the establishment of such plans. Indeed, under rulings of the National Labor Relations Board, employers are required to bargain in good faith with their employees, not only over hours and wages, but also in regard to their pension plan.

In recent years, further steps have been taken by Congress to encourage the growth of private pensions. The self-employed have been able, since the 1950s, to establish their own retirement plans. Even persons working for others have been able to set up their own Individual Retirement Accounts (IRAs) to supplement Social Security benefits in retirement. The tax reform legislation of 1981 made it possible for any person to set up an IRA whether or not that person is included in a private pension plan of an employer.

With the establishment of the SSI program, the federal government finally tackled the difficult problem of minimum adequacy. In 2005, the federal government assured the aged of $579 income per month ($869 for a couple living together) (Social Security Administration, 2004a). This amount could consist of an SSI supplement to Social Security or other income, or it could all be the SSI payment. The figures given above are indexed to the cost of living and are adjusted annually, as are basic Social Security benefits. At the end of 2003, 7 million individuals were receiving SSI checks with an average value of $417 per month. Of these 7 million recipients, more than 1 million were over the age of 65 (Social Security Administration, 2004b). Unfortunately, despite its availability only half of all individuals eligible for SSI were receiving it in 2000 (Herd, 2005).

Old-Age Benefits

The entire Social Security program is work related. Individuals are eligible for benefits only if they have been in employment (or self-employment) or are dependent upon one who has been so employed. Specific requirements concerning the length of employment and the kind of work must be met in order to qualify for benefits. The basic requirements for Social Security are the same for all programs—old-age benefits, survivor's benefits, and disability benefits—and are only slightly modified for medical benefits. The basic requirement involves 40 quarters, or 10 years, of work in "covered employment." In 2006, an income of $970 earned an employee a quarter's credit Social Security. Any income below this level was not counted in the employee's Social Security record (Social Security Administration, 2005).

The 40 quarters that are needed in order to be eligible for Social Security can be accumulated over a period of a lifetime. "Covered employment" has been broadly defined to include all work performed as an employee in commerce or industry or in self-employment. Work in certain government operations or nonprofit organizations is also included if a particular agreement has been made between the federal government and these other levels of government or nonprofit employers.

Workers covered by Social Security pay a tax on their earnings, and employers add a like amount. The size of the ultimate benefit is based on a calculation that takes into account the total of such taxable earnings. When the system was first initiated in 1936, the maximum earnings subject to tax were $3,000 a year. Over the years, this amount has gradually been increased. In 1979, the taxable earnings base was $22,900. The ceiling on earnings subject to tax was $94,200 in 2006. People whose annual incomes are in excess of these amounts pay taxes only on the first $94,200 they earn. When the taxable base is increased, it affects only those workers who have been earning more than the previous year's taxable base (Pear, 2005).

The tax rate is also fixed by law. In 2006, the tax rate was 7.65% of the first $94,200 of an individual's earnings. Of this amount, 6.2% is allotted for Social Security and disability insurance; the remainder is for Medicare (Social Security Administration, 2005). The tax rate for the self-employed is now equivalent to that paid by the salaried worker and employer. This change, however, did not come fully into effect until 1990. Self-employed persons pay their Social Security tax each year at the same time as they pay their federal income tax (U.S. House of Representatives, 1991). There are no maximum taxable earnings for Medicare.

Veterans receive gratuitous credit for military service between September 1940 and December 1957. When veterans apply for benefits, it is assumed that they earned $160 per month during their years of military service. After 1957, servicemen paid the Social Security tax on their military earnings and therefore are eligible for benefits the same as any other employed person.

The size of the benefits reflects the level of earnings during the wage earner's working years. When a wage earner applies for benefits, lifetime earnings, that is, earnings from age 21 until the time of application, are totaled. The five lowest years of earnings are excluded, and the number of months—less the excluded five years—is divided into the total earnings. The resulting amount—the Average Monthly Earnings—is then plotted against a table provided in the law to determine the monthly benefit that will be received. The table of benefits reflects some favorable treatment for low-paid workers in that they receive more in benefits as a proportion of previous earnings than do higher-paid workers.

Without any action by the Congress, benefits are automatically adjusted annually to reflect changes in the cost of living. Inasmuch as Social Security benefits are only partially subject to income tax, this adjustment enables beneficiaries to maintain their purchasing power under the pressures of upward movement of prices (inflation). Until this procedure became automatic, an act of Congress was necessary to adjust benefits. The Cost of Living Adjustment was 4.1 percent in 2006 (Pear, 2005).

The average monthly Social Security benefit in 2006 was $1,002 (Pear, 2005). There is, however, a maximum benefit allowed, which was $2,053 per month in 2006 (Social Security Administration, 2005). There is no longer any minimum benefit for workers except for beneficiaries already on the rolls. There is still a one-time death benefit of $255 for survivors.

Because Social Security is calculated on the worker's wages, low-income workers also receive lower benefits than higher-income workers. The law now provides that long-term low-paid workers will receive benefits larger than they would under the normal formula incorporated in the law. Social Security replaces about 70% of the income of workers who earned $10,000 a year, but only replaces 28.5% of the income of those who earned over $70,000 per year (Andrews, 2005).

Social Security has become a vital component of retirement income for older persons. It makes up more than half of the income of two-thirds of all individuals over the age of 65. For 22% of beneficiaries, Social Security is their only source of income (Pear, 2005).

Until 2000, the age for full retirement benefits was 65. Workers who have the required number of quarters of coverage can retire at an age as low as 62. The benefits for these earners are reduced on an actuarial basis so that their early retirement does not cost the system any money. This reduction is 20% for those retiring at age 62, proportionately less as the individual nears age 65 when applying for benefits. More than half of current applications for retirement benefits are being made by persons who are below 65 years of age. The age at which an individual can collect full benefits will gradually rise over the next 30 years. For individuals born between 1943 and 1954, the age for full benefits will be 66. For individuals born in 1960 and later, the full age for eligibility will be 67.

The benefits of a retired wage earner may be increased if his or her spouse is of the appropriate age. This provision was added to the law in 1939 at a time when the pattern of family living was for the husband to be in gainful employment to support his spouse and children. The 50% increase in the wage earner's benefits was on behalf of the wife who had not been employed outside the home. That addendum is paid in the instances of spouses who have no earning records of their own, or in cases where a spouse's earning record would yield a benefit of a lesser amount than she (or he) would receive as a dependent spouse. The Social Security Administration will make a comparison at the time of application for benefits and award the larger of the two amounts. Although the addendum is added to the wage earner's monthly check, the wife can receive a separate check if she requests it. An addendum is also allowable if the retired wage earner has dependent children living at home. In this instance, benefits are payable on behalf of such children up to the age of 18, unless the children are full-time elementary or secondary students.

The law provides, however, that if the husband or wife who is claiming benefits on the basis of the earnings of the other is also receiving benefits from any governmental program, the spouse's benefits will be reduced by the amount of the additional benefit being received. The purpose of this provision is to disallow the Social Security benefits claimed by a spouse who is covered by the U.S. Civil Service retirement system or a comparable state system and who consequently is not in any way dependent upon the spouse who is covered by Social Security.

In the past, benefits were payable to retired wage earners if they met the retirement test as stated in the law. The test of retirement was in terms of annual earnings. Individuals receiving Social Security benefits but also earning an annual amount higher than the amount stated in the law lost part or, if the earnings are sufficiently large, all of their benefits. In 1996, Congress voted to raise the earnings limit and in 2000 legislation repealed the earning test. This means that individuals can now work and earn unlimited income without losing any of their Social Security benefits.

A common problem experienced by older people involves the death of a spouse and the remarriage of the surviving spouse who receives Social Security benefits. Often, the remarriage is to a person who also receives benefits. A spouse who receives survivor's benefits could lose them upon remarriage. As a result of amendments to the law that became effective in 1979, the remarriage of a surviving spouse after age 60 will not reduce the amount of benefits.

Another problem occurs in the breakup of a marriage that leaves a divorced mate without any marriage ties to a retired worker and thus unable to claim the spouse's 50% addendum. A divorced spouse who was married for 10 years may claim benefits based on the former spouse's earning record at the time of retirement. The fact that the wage earner may have remarried does not affect the benefits to the divorced spouse. Prior to 1983, the divorced spouse was in a difficult position if he or she did not have an earning record and the former spouse chose to continue working. Under the 1983 amendments to the Act, the divorced spouse can now collect Social Security benefits at age 62, regardless of whether or not the former spouse applies for his or her own benefits.

FINANCING SOCIAL SECURITY

The financial integrity of the Social Security system is of crucial importance to its beneficiaries. All costs of the program, including the cost of administering it, come from a tax imposed on employers and employees. This tax money is identified separately in the United States Treasury and is available for appropriation to pay benefits and the cost of administration. Although most wage earners believe the Social Security tax is a single figure, it is actually a series of smaller tax sums designed to reflect the cost of the various elements of the system. These include the retirement program, disability, survivors, and health insurance. In recent years, it has become apparent that some of these so-called trust funds for individual program purposes were running short and soon would be in deficit. The 1983 amendments, which increased both the tax base and the tax rate, rescued the Social Security system from imminent deficit. The amendments increased the flow of money into the Treasury from wage earners and employers and thus gave assurance that, for at least a time, the income was equal to the outgo.

Because the Social Security system is financed solely by the tax on employers and employees, there is no other money from the Treasury going into the basic system. Unless the nation should decide to allocate some general revenue funds to pay at least part of the costs, the benefits will continue to be paid for by the payroll tax.

The problems of Social Security are both short-range and long-range. In the short range, sluggish economic activity (which reduces the number of employee contributors as a consequence of unemployment) and inflation (which requires an upward adjustment in benefits) can put a strain on the money needed for payments to beneficiaries. In the long run, the growing number of aged in the population and the reduction in the working-age population means that a reduced proportion of younger people will be supporting an increasing proportion of older people.

In 1983, under the pressures of keeping the Social Security system solvent, a bipartisan commission developed proposals that were signed into law. As already noted, the 1983 amendments set new tax rates and salary bases. These increases are designed to bring additional money into the system and offset the increasing number of beneficiaries and the cost-of-living adjustments to which they are now entitled.

Besides requiring individuals already paying Social Security taxes to pay more, the 1983 amendments also tried to use two other strategies to shore up the Social Security trust fund: (1) increase the number of individuals paying the taxes, and (2) encourage people to retire later and thus continue to pay into the system for a longer period.

For the first strategy, the 1983 amendments required all new federal workers to pay Social Security taxes. This change added a significant pool of new taxpayers who formerly paid into a separate federal civil service system. Any local and state governments currently covered by the Social Security system were now forbidden to withdraw from the system in order to set up their own retirement plans.

One element of the strategy to encourage people to work longer was the dismantling of the earning tests. Even more important was the raise in the age of retirement with full benefits. Individuals who do not apply for their benefits when they reach the full age of retirement will also be rewarded with higher benefit levels when they receive their benefits. For example, individuals who retire at 67 will receive 8% more benefits for each year they delay in collecting these benefits (e.g., 108% at age 68, 116% at age 69).

At least one group of beneficiaries, however, has found that the 1983 amendments did not necessarily provide them with any increase in their total income. Half of Social Security benefits are now counted as taxable income for individuals whose gross income combined with Social Security benefits exceeds $25,000 ($32,000 for a married couple). For single individuals with income over $34,000 ($44,000 for a married couple), 85% of their benefits are taxable. The counting of Social Security benefits as taxable income is a major departure from past practices. Importantly, the funds derived from these taxes are contributed to the Social Security trust funds as a means of further ensuring its solvency.

SURVIVOR'S INSURANCE

Benefits for survivors of deceased wage earners under the Social Security system are available to the survivors (wife or husband and young children) of a prematurely deceased wage earner. These benefits are also available to the surviving spouse (age 60 or older and younger children of any) of a wage earner who was either retired or had been eligible for retirement. For purposes of this chapter, only the latter group of survivors—the older people—will be discussed.

As explained earlier, an addendum will be added to the benefit of a spouse if he or she is at least 60 years of age. This benefit is paid not only on behalf of spouses who have had no employment record of their own. Individuals who worked in covered employment but for whom the earned benefit is less than 50% of the wage earner's Primary Insurance Amount (PIA) are also covered. The survivor's benefit is 100% of the wage earner's PIA. Thus it is possible for a woman whose earned benefit was less than 50% of her husband's to receive a larger benefit upon the death of her husband. A benefit of the same size will also be paid to the widow or widower of a wage earner who had been eligible for a retirement benefit but who had not claimed it. In the event the aged survivor also has responsibility for young children of the deceased, the benefit will be 75% of the PIA plus a payment made on behalf of each child equal to 75% of the PIA. Benefits are also payable to dependent parents of deceased wage earners.

Beneficiaries of survivor's benefits are subject to the same earnings test as are retired people. Therefore, if a widower or widow is employed and receiving an income, the survivor's benefit might be reduced or even eliminated, depending on the amount of the survivor's earnings.

SUPPLEMENTARY SECURITY INCOME

The SSI program was established in 1974 on the basis of legislation enacted in 1972. It provides for federalizing the former grants-in-aid programs of old-age assistance, aid to the blind, and aid to the permanently and totally disabled. Except for the disability component, these programs had been administered by the states since 1935, with states administering grants for the disabled since 1950. Under the 1972 legislation, the federal government provides assistance to the aged, blind, and disabled who qualify under the specific provisions of the law. National standards are used both for eligibility and for payment.

There are several major differences between the SSI program and the comparable old-age and disability programs in the Social Security system. Unlike Social Security, the SSI program is means-tested. Funds for the SSI program come from the general revenue of the Treasury, whereas Social Security is financed by a payroll tax on employers and employees. The SSI program is available to anyone who meets the qualifications of age, blindness, and disability, without regard to participation in the workforce. The

Social Security program is directly related to employment, either by the beneficiary or by his or her dependents. Although both Social Security and SSI are administered by the Social Security Administration, a distinction is maintained between the two programs.

National eligibility requirements for SSI are:

- Inmates of public institutions are not eligible.
- The payments to eligible individuals living in a medical institution such as a nursing home are reduced to $30 per month.
- If individuals do not apply for other benefits for which they are eligible, such as Social Security, they cannot receive an SSI payment.
- Individuals with substance abuse problems can receive payments only if they are in a treatment program approved by the federal government and in compliance with the treatment plan.
- Individuals living outside the United States are not eligible for SSI.
- Disabled persons under the age of 65 must accept a referral to the state vocational rehabilitation agency for a study of their condition and must accept a proposed plan of treatment in order to continue eligibility for SSI.
- Applicants must be either citizens or legally admitted aliens in order to be eligible for SSI.
- Persons who are age 65, or blind, or disabled are eligible. If the eligibility is blindness or disability, the individual must meet the test used in the Social Security program of disability insurance.
- The resources of an eligible individual must not exceed $2,000 and $3,000 for a couple.

The system promises a certain level of income, which consists of SSI alone, if the individual has no other income, or a combination of SSI and other income to reach the established payment level. In determining the amount an individual or a couple will receive, some modifications are made in the treatment of income:

- Only net income from employment is counted. Income includes earnings, cash, checks, and in-kind income such as food and shelter.
- The first $240 per year of income such as from Social Security is not counted, but all income paid on the basis of need is fully counted.
- Earned income of eligible persons up to $780 per year is not counted.
- Casual and inconsequential income not to exceed $60 in a quarter is not counted.

- If the eligible individual is living in another person's household and is receiving support or maintenance in kind, the SSI payment is reduced by one-third.

In 2005 an individual could have an income of up to $579 a month and still be eligible for SSI, and a couple could have an income of up to $861 per month. With its complex system of "disregards," it is possible for an individual to have an income of up to $1,211 and still receive SSI benefits (Social Security Administration, 2004c).

A state may establish a higher payment level at its own expense but may not add eligibility requirements. The federal government will administer that payment at no administrative cost to the state. Many states have chosen to provide a state supplement, with some states administering it themselves. This means that the payment level varies around the country as individual states decide whether to add to the federal payment, how much to add, and to what extent these supplements should be increased as living costs rise. In FY 1998, there were more than 1.4 million individuals receiving SSI on the basis of age out of a total of 6.5 million recipients (Social Security Administration, n.d.).

STATE GENERAL ASSISTANCE PROGRAMS

Many states have a program of general assistance that is the direct linear descendant of the old poor law relief programs. Like these earlier programs, they are largely local in character. Some states, however, help finance the program and may even set state standards. The primary eligibility provision is need, which is often severely tested.

This program is available to persons who do not qualify for other programs such as Social Security and SSI. A likely candidate, for example, is a needy person aged 60. Unless such persons are disabled or blind, they would not be eligible for Social Security or SSI and could very well be in need. Inasmuch as there is no federal financial help in the state programs, the availability of benefits depends upon state eligibility requirements and often some local requirements. During the early 1990s, General Assistance programs in many states suffered major cuts as the recession reduced state revenues; in some states they have been eliminated completely.

PRIVATE PENSION PLANS

Private pensions are becoming an increasingly large part of the national income support system. As noted earlier, the federal government has encouraged and facilitated their development. Although looking favorably on these programs, the federal government finds it difficult to impose effective controls over them. The reason is that, fundamentally, these are private programs, and the federal government cannot readily make demands about what industry and commerce do with their private programs.

By 1974, however, several situations had developed in private pension plans that forced the federal government to take action. Evidence was accumulating that there was gross inequity in the benefits being paid. There were indications of corruption by managers of the plans. Poorly funded plans were being set up, which, in all probability, would not be able to pay benefits. Meanwhile, workers were making retirement plans under the expectation of receiving benefits from their private pension plans to supplement what they knew would be inadequate Social Security benefits.

The private sector has a choice of whether or not it wants to provide a pension plan, and it retains the choice of discontinuing a plan once one is set up. The benefit rights of an individual are only rarely transferable when the worker moves from one employer to another. Social Security remains the only income support insurance program with that feature.

The main objective of the federal legislation was to assure the receipt of benefits upon retirement after a period of service for an employer. Setting up a reinsurance fund, similar to the Federal Deposit Insurance Corporation (which insures bank deposits), provided a further assurance. The reinsurance fund collects a small fee from all pension funds and maintains a reserve to pay off accumulated obligations to beneficiaries of any bankrupt fund.

The standards imposed by federal law on the private pensions operate separately for funds in which the employee has contributed as compared to those in which the employer makes all the contributions. There are more severe requirements for vesting (the rights to a benefit) for the former than for the latter. For the employer-financed funds, vesting the benefits takes place following 5 years of service. After that time, the benefit payment to which the employee is entitled grows as the number of years employed, when added to the employee's age, becomes larger. Conceivably, an employee could work for several companies, working the minimum number of years for each, in order to have vested rights and, upon retirement, receive several benefit checks, although each would be a small one.

Vesting can be accomplished in two ways. Under "cliff vesting" funds are 100% vested after 10 years. This is reduced to 5 years for individuals hired after 1989. Under "graded vesting" 25% of the funds are vested after 5 years. The percentage of the contributions vested increases until 100% is vested after 15 years. As is true of "cliff vesting," graded vesting for employees hired after 1989 begins at 3 years (25% vested) and is completed after 7 years.

There are several important characteristics of the private pension system:

- The payments are growing in adequacy, although they do not equal those of Social Security. An exception is benefits to high-level executives, who often have a generous pension plan built into their remuneration.
- Benefits are payable to survivors of deceased plan members in a small but slowly growing number of plans.
- Few plans provide for adjustment to the cost of living, and if they do, it is not usually the full increase.
- The plans tend to favor the long-term employee, who, by virtue of continuous employment by one employer, can become eligible for a more significant payment.
- In a few instances, an employee may carry over benefit rights to another employer in the same industry. An example is the trucker's pension fund, which operates across the industry.

Private pension funds share the same problem of nearly all retirement plans in the United States: they are marginally secure financially. The insurance fund accumulates reserves very slowly and could be wiped out by a few large claims made simultaneously. The actuarially determined obligation for pension payments on some corporations, even large corporations, is excessive. One issue that will gradually have to be faced is the extent of the corporate obligation for payment under terms of the plan versus the shareholders' rights to the assets of the company. If corporations encounter difficult economic times, they may also reconsider their involvement in an extensive pension effort.

The Insurance and Public Benefits section of the 1992 Older Americans Act amendments (Title VII) is supposed to help older workers evaluate the pension plans in which they are enrolled or for which they are eligible. The aim of this state-run program is to help older individuals understand the ability of these pensions to meet their post-retirement needs and the relationship of these pensions to other public benefits and insurance plans. Although it is likely that this issue will be resolved without reaching a crunch, it does suggest that the private pension system has to face the reality of financing troubles.

Individual Retirement Accounts (IRAs) are one alternative for individuals who do not have private pension plans available. The interest on these accounts in banks, mutual funds, or insurance companies is not taxable until the individual withdraws the funds between the ages of 59½ and 70. Earlier withdrawal is subject to major penalties on the interest. Under the Tax Relief Act of 1997, individuals with an adjusted gross income of

$30,000, and couples with an adjusted gross income of $50,000, can contribute $2,000 worth of deductible income into an IRA each year. Individuals with an adjusted gross income of $95,000 ($150,000 for couples) can contribute $2,000 after-tax income to an IRA. These funds must stay in the IRA for at least 5 years and are not taxed when they are withdrawn from the IRA.

Although pension reform has been extensive, there are still major differences in the proportion of minority and non-minority workers who are covered by pensions. In 2002, 33% of White workers, 24% of African American workers, and 14% of Latino workers were covered by pensions (Wu, 2004). These changes probably represent some loss of opportunities for minority workers to obtain jobs where pension coverage is offered as well as the increase in voluntary salary reduction plans. Among workers offered these voluntary plans, White workers have a higher rate of participation than others. These differences in pension coverage rates will mean that more minority older persons than before will have to rely on Social Security to meet their financial needs after they retire.

In order to fully evaluate the adequacy of the income available to older persons it is necessary to assess all of the sources of income they are able to draw upon. Although 89% of individuals over the age of 65 had Social Security coverage in 2002, only 30% were covered by pensions with a median income from these pensions of $8,400. In addition, 53% of older individuals had some income from interest but this interest amounted to only a median figure of $600 per year. Finally, 16.3% had some work related earnings with a median value of $15,000 per year (Wu, 2004).

These figures clearly indicate the continuing importance of Social Security income for many older individuals. The reliance on Social Security is even stronger among minority elders because, as already noted, they are less likely to have private pensions. In addition, although 59% of White elderly have some income from interest this is true of only 24% of Black elderly and 22% of Latino elderly. The differences in income from dividends is even more marked: 26% of White elderly have some dividend income, but this form of income is available to only 5% of Black elderly and 6% of Latino elderly (Wu, 2004).

UNEMPLOYMENT AND INADEQUATE INCOME

The distinction between unemployment of an older person and retirement is often a thin one. Older people who lose their jobs may be vigorously looking for other ones; yet, because they need income, they may be forced to apply for and accept some income transfer benefits. Before moving on to the Social Security program, these people may wish to exhaust their unemployment compensation rights. Many older persons receive unemployment compensation, either before moving on to Social Security or simultaneously. It is possible for a person to receive both unemployment compensation and old-age benefits at the same time.

Unemployment compensation is a program of benefits for persons who were employed in specified fields of work but who have, not of their own choosing, left their jobs. The program is administered by the states, which have considerable latitude in establishing eligibility standards, including the amount of the weekly benefit. Unemployment compensation is financed by a federally imposed tax, most of which is returned to the states by the federal government to pay the cost of the benefits granted and the cost of administering the program, which includes the operation of an employment service. States may add to the amount of the tax, making more funds available to support more generous benefits. States may also increase the duration of benefits and pay the cost of less onerous provisions for eligibility. Many states do this.

The number of workers covered by unemployment compensation has been increasing in recent years, until most workers in commerce and industry and many people in public employment and in teaching professions are now covered. Some progress has been made in incorporating casual employment, such as domestic and farm work, into the system. Even so, most people engaged in these kinds of jobs are still not covered, nor are self-employed persons. Benefits are payable only after a worker has been in employment for a specified period of time set by the states and therefore varying from state to state, with 26 weeks emerging as the most common length of time.

The trend has been for Congress to provide extended benefits in the course of an economic recession. The receipt of benefits has extended for as long as 15 months in recent years, but duration of more than 9 months is no longer likely. Many people question the wisdom of these extensions on the grounds that the availability of benefits tends to discourage diligent search for work. Such a long period of unemployment also strongly indicates that a work program is needed rather than an income transfer program. If benefits are to be extended, many observers contend, the recipients of such benefits ought to be means-tested, which they are not now. Some unemployment benefits are subject to income tax. Some states include an addendum for dependents, but generally benefits are awarded to the worker without regard for family circumstances.

Eligibility for benefits hinges upon the unemployed individual being ready, willing, and able to work. Presumably, illness or disability should exclude a worker, although in practice the unavailability of the worker for a job often is not known to the state. An unemployed person is not expected to take the first job that materializes without regard to experi-ence or training; the system allows workers to hold off accepting em-ployment until a job becomes available that uses their skills. As time passes, however, unemployed workers are expected to lower their job ex-pectations and accept less ideal work. Workers are not expected to take strike-breaking jobs or jobs that offer below the usual wages.

Workers who wish to receive unemployment compensation are re-quired to register for work with the employment service. If that office is successful in finding a job for the recipient of unemployment compensa-tion, the unemployed person is expected to accept it, unless he or she can show good cause for not doing so. Inasmuch as the employment service has few job openings for older workers, it is unlikely that an older per-son's willingness to work will be put to a test. Even if the employment of-fice should refer the unemployment compensation beneficiary to a job, the employer may reject him or her, and this would not affect continued eligibility for benefits.

The basic program of unemployment compensation benefits is sometimes supplemented by private funds created as a consequence of labor–management agreements. In the automobile, steel, and some other highly organized industries, management contributes toward a fund used to supplement the basic unemployment compensation program whenever needed. This supplement can take the form of continuing benefits after the regular program ends or, more likely, can supplement the size of the basic benefit. These funds are relatively new, having been established only in recent years. When put to a test, they were proven to be insufficient to last the duration of the unemployment period in the industries, although they were helpful to the workers who received them. These supplementary funds tend to provide more help to those with the greatest job seniority.

REFERENCES

Andrews, E. (2005, March 20). G.O.P. courts Blacks and Hispanics on Social Security. *New York Times*, p. A21.

Herd, P. (2005). Ensuring a minimum: Social Security reform and women. *The Gerontologist, 45,* 12–25.

Pear, R. (2005, October 15). Benefit rising by 4 percent, but Medicare takes a share. *New York Times*, p. A15.

Social Security Administration. (n.d.). *Social Security online: Management of the Supplemental Security Income Program.* Retrieved November 18, 2005, from http://www.ssa.gov/reports/ssi/intro.htm

Social Security Administration. (2004a). *Automatic increases: SSI federal pay-ment amounts.* Retrieved December 16, 2004, from http://www.ssa.gov/OACT/COLA/SSI.html

Social Security Administration. (2004b). *Monthly statistical snapshot: September, 2004*. Retrieved October 18, 2004, from http://www.ssa.gov/policy/docs/quickfacts/stat_snapshot/

Social Security Administration. (2004c). *Social Security online: Answers to your questions*. Retrieved October 20, 2004, from http://ssa-custhelp.ssa.gov/

Social Security Administration. (2005). *Social Security online: Answers to your questions*. Retrieved October 18, 2005, from http://ssa-custhelp.ssa.gov/

U.S. House of Representatives, Committee on Ways and Means. (1991). *Background material and data on programs within the jurisdiction of the Committee on Ways and Means*. Washington, DC: U.S. Government Printing Office.

Wu, K. (2004). *Sources of income for older persons in 2002*. AARP Public Policy Institute. Retrieved December 6, 2004, from http://research.aarp.org/econ/dd/04_income.pdf

CHAPTER FOUR

Illness, Medical Care, and Income Maintenance

Becoming ill or disabled creates two major problems for those affected. The first problem can be a loss of income because of an inability to work. ①
The second is how to pay for needed medical care. ②

RISKS OF ILLNESS, DISABILITY, AND INADEQUATE INCOME

Several programs, all of which depend on the particular status of the individual, address the need for income. Although older individuals are usually eligible for the federally funded Medicare program, a substantial number of workers are forced to retire at earlier ages because of disability. The Social Security program includes benefits available to persons disabled on a long-term basis. Some states provide short-term disability benefits as an element in their unemployment compensation program. Worker's compensation is available for those who have become ill or disabled on the job; this includes wage replacement and medical expenses. Many employers provide sick leave, which is a form of short-term disability benefit. The SSI program is available for the disabled who, for one reason or another, are not eligible for Social Security or any other income-producing programs.

Social Security Disability Benefits

Eligibility for Social Security benefits generally follows along the lines of eligibility for Social Security in general, as described in Chapter 3. The major difference in eligibility between the two programs is a requirement for a longer attachment to the labor force. Although disability benefits are available to younger workers who meet the test of severity of disability, the law requires disabled persons to have worked under covered employment for a proportionately longer period of time than is required of deceased wage earners who die prematurely and leave survivors. The intention is to emphasize that the worker to be covered has made a significant financial contribution to the system before becoming eligible.

For purposes of determining the amount of benefits after disabled workers establish eligibility on the basis of severity of disability and length of time in the workforce, they are considered retired. Their lifetime wages in covered employment are totaled and divided by the number of months of work. For younger workers, the number of months of covered employment may be small, certainly when compared to those of the retired person. However, the average monthly earnings of the younger worker could be as high as those of a retired worker. Indeed, the monthly average might well be higher, as the younger worker's wage history s more recent and covers a time when wages have been higher than those of a retired person whose wage history may go back 40 years. This peculiarity of the system has resulted in disability benefits generally running higher than those granted for retired persons.

Legislation enacted in 1980 set some ceilings on benefits for the disabled in order to ensure that benefits do not exceed previous earnings but reduce the gap between retirement and disability benefits. Benefits for disabled workers are increased if they have spouses and even more if they have dependent children. The procedure for determining the amount of these awards is similar to that used for retired workers, their spouses, and their young children, if any.

For claiming benefits, the definition of disability is a severe one. It attempts to limit the program to those persons with severe and long-lasting disabilities, either mental or physical. The words in the definition, "inability to engage in any substantial gainful activity," suggest that a test is to be made of the individual's ability to engage in "any gainful activity," not just a test of whether or not there is employment in the community in which the individual lives. This definition could conceivably result in the denial of benefits to people who might be able to do certain kinds of work even if there was no possibility of any work of that nature showing up.

The individual applicant is responsible for presenting proof of disability and, if medical examination or testing is involved, must pay for that cost. If the Social Security Administration is not satisfied with the proof offered, it will pay for additionally required examinations and reports.

Although the definition speaks in terms of long and severe disability, from the very beginning the assumption has been that some beneficiaries might be rehabilitated. For this reason, provision is made for each state's vocational rehabilitation agency to review all applications with a view toward identification of potential cases for vocational rehabilitation. Applicants who are recommended by the agency for rehabilitation must accept the plan of that agency or forfeit their rights to disability benefits. In some instances, the rehabilitation plan is financed by the Social Security Administration as a charge against Social Security funds. Those who are rehabilitated and who go off the program save the program a great deal of money over the years.

The cost of rehabilitation is usually regarded as a prudent investment. The actual record of rehabilitation cases shows that comparatively few applicants are able to be fully rehabilitated and return to work. Legislation under consideration would encourage beneficiaries to undertake work by assuring them of quick reentry to the program if the work does not prove feasible.

Under heightened review processes, an increased number of individuals receiving disability payments were terminated during the early 1980s. This included many older individuals who had received disability payments for many years. In fiscal 1983, the benefits of 182,074 workers were terminated, as compared to 80,956 in 1981 (U.S. House of Representatives, 1986). In response to mounting complaints about unjust terminations, the law now provides the individual with the right to a face-to-face hearing before benefits are terminated. Appeals procedures have also been clarified. The Disabilities Reform Act of 1984 specified the reasons for termination of disability benefits, including standards of medical improvement.

Sick Leave

Important, but often overlooked, resources for providing income to people who are temporarily sick or disabled are the provisions many employers make for sick leave. Employers who provide sick leave tend to be those who employ white-collar workers. However, manufacturing companies have begun to provide this benefit as well. Government work of all kinds includes this form of illness protection. A specific and very important form of leave is now provided through the Family and Medical Leave Act enacted by Congress in 1993. Under this law, an employee is eligible for unpaid leave for up to 12 weeks within a 12-month period to care for newborn children or to care for a spouse, child, or parent with a serious health problem. A parent is defined as a biological parent or an individual who was "in loco parentis" when the employee was a child, but not an in-law.

Worker's Compensation

The states, or private insurance companies under state supervision, operate programs of worker's compensation. Typically, benefits include both financial assistance in lieu of lost wages and payment for medical bills.

The illnesses and disabilities covered by this program are those incurred on the job, under the concept of no-fault; that is, no test is made to determine whether employees were careless or otherwise contributed to their own accidents. Benefits are often time limited and are usually related to the severity of the disability. For the severely disabled, benefits include some form of rehabilitation, often in conjunction with the state vocational rehabilitation agency.

Not all employees are covered by worker's compensation. Because these are state programs, eligibility provisions differ around the country. In some states there are exemptions of small employers, usually defined as those with five employees. Typically, other employees not covered are domestic, casual, and farm workers. Because of these variations among the states and omissions from the program, there is some interest in enacting a federal law that would establish uniform standards for the nation.

Temporary Disability Insurance

Short-term disability benefits are available in some states as an offshoot of the unemployment insurance program. These states include some of the large industrial states, such as New York and California.

Benefits are available for workers who are covered by the state unemployment insurance law and who are absent from work because of illness or disability. These are people whose illness or disability is unrelated to their work (otherwise, they would be eligible for worker's compensation) and whose absence from work will be temporary, as contrasted with the long-term absences defined in the Social Security program. Workers covered by an employer's sick leave may not be excluded in some states; in others, disability benefits may be reduced or denied. Temporary disability benefits are not permitted to overlap unemployment insurance benefit payments.

All of the laws have minimum requirements for days absent or loss of wages before benefits will begin and, of course, set limits on the duration of the benefit being paid. Benefits are related to the size of previous earnings, as in the case of unemployment compensation. The plans are financed by a state-imposed tax on employees and, in some states, on the employers. There is no federal financial support for these programs.

RISKS OF AGING, MEDICAL BILLS, AND INADEQUATE INCOME

In 2003, U.S. spending for health care accounted for 15% of the gross domestic product. Between 2002 and 2003, total health spending increased by 7.7%. In addition, premiums for private health care insurance increased 9.3% in 2003. These increases are reflected in the fact that health care spending in the United States reached an average of $5,670 per person in 2003.

The increase in health care costs was also reflected in Medicare, the major payer of health care costs for older persons, reaching $283 billion, an increase of 5.7% from 2002 (Pear, 2005a). As the number of older individuals increases and new drugs and technologies become available, continued increases in health care expenditures can be expected. For these reasons, provisions to help the aged meet medical costs have been in the law for many years. From the earliest history of government and through the years, welfare programs have provided some medical care and some payment for medical care for poor people, especially the aged. That practice is now being carried out through the Medicaid program.

Private insurance for health care costs has been available for decades, but has been especially prominent since World War II. The Blue Cross plan for hospital insurance was begun during the Depression and has had many individual and group subscribers. Private health insurance has become a fringe benefit of employment. While Blue Cross as a nonprofit community plan had a large number of old persons as subscribers, other private plans (especially the profit-making ones) shunned the elderly because of their poor risk record, and conducted all of their business through employers. Thus, if older persons remained in employment, they would have some financial help for medical expenses in this manner.

It became obvious over time that private health insurance could not be depended upon to provide protection for the aged. Indeed, there was doubt that private profit-making health insurance companies wanted a major role in insuring them. The high incidence of illness among the aged made them a poor risk for private health insurance. Although private Blue Cross plans have been an exception to this rule, even this group of nonprofit private insurers began to be concerned about the stability of their financial position, especially as the cost of hospital care began to escalate dramatically in the 1960s. Even though the private health insurance industry and private medical practitioners were opposed to further government involvement, the public interest and demand for hospital insurance for the aged prevailed, and Medicare was enacted in 1965.

Private programs vary widely in the protection offered, provisions for coverage, and circumstances of enrollment, but provide considerable protection for many older persons, especially those under the age of 65. For those over age 65, private health insurance is widely available to supplement the Medicare program. Medicare covers nearly all persons age 65 and over, those receiving disability benefits under Social Security, and a few other small groups. Eligibility and benefits will be discussed below.

As the older population has continued to increase and the number of workers decrease, the problem of financing Medicare looms larger. One projection is that the hospital trust fund for Part A of Medicare will be in a crisis situation when individual baby boomers become eligible for Medicare in 2008. This date is partly based on projections that the number of workers paying into Medicare will drop to 2.8 by 2020 and to 2.2 by 2040. There are also projections that unless birth rates change, by the year 2040 only 2.2 workers will pay into Medicare for every one beneficiary (Federal Hospital Insurance Trust Fund, 1998). In 2005, the trustees of the Medicare program predicted that Medicare funds would be depleted by 2014 (Rosenbaum, 2005). To combat this likelihood, changes have been discussed in taxes paid for Medicare, deductibles, and premiums paid by beneficiaries. The federal balanced budget bill passed in 1997 reduced reimbursements to hospitals and physicians but some of these cuts have been restored.

To control hospital costs, a new system of prospective payment for hospital care has been introduced. This Diagnostic Related Group (DRG) system uses standardized payments for particular conditions. The results of this system have been controversial. Some critics have argued that older patients are being discharged prematurely. The Medicare Quality Protection Act of 1986 required hospitals to prepare discharge plans for patients who might be adversely affected by discharge. Patients must also be informed of their rights to inpatient hospitalization and have the right to appeal a decision for discharging them. By 1989, hospital stays for persons over age 65 had declined to 8.9 days (National Center for Health Statistics, 1991). In contrast to the federally controlled Medicare program, Medicaid is a grant-in-aid program operated by the states and provides protection for some of the poor population. Coverage varies from state to state, and benefits also vary, but are broader than those of Medicare. The differences can be seen through a discussion of both Medicare and Medicaid.

Medicare

Medicare is an integral part of the Social Security program. Generally speaking, eligibility for Medicare is determined by eligibility for Social Security; Medicare benefits are provided to persons who have established eligibility for old-age benefits or disability benefits. No separate eligibility determination is made except for disabled beneficiaries, who must have been in receipt of cash benefits for 2 years prior to Medicare eligibility. Medicare is not available to persons who are below the age of 65, except for individuals suffering from end-stage renal disease or who are disabled.

The Medicare program is divided into two parts: Part A—hospital insurance—and Part B—medical insurance. All persons eligible for Medicare receive Part A benefits without any additional cost to them. Part B benefits are available only to persons who "join," that is, agree to pay a certain amount each month. This monthly fee is deducted from the checks of persons who receive Social Security cash benefits. In the case of persons who are eligible for Social Security benefits but who do not receive a check because they are earning above the retirement level, a bill from Medicare is sent for subsequent payment. In both parts, deductibles and coinsurance payments are required.

Part A

Under Part A, persons with a medically established need for hospitalization are entitled to 60 days of hospitalization. As a condition of eligibility, they must pay a premium of $206 and a set amount for the first 60 days of care. That amount is raised annually as the cost of hospitalization increases. It was $952 in 2006. If additional days of hospital care are needed, 30 more days are available upon the payment of a daily coinsurance fee, which in 2006 was $238. This fee is also raised annually. There must be a short period of time between hospitalizations before the 60-day and 30-day periods become applicable again. If additional hospitalization is needed beyond the 60- and 30-day limits, an individual can draw upon a lifetime reserve allowable for each eligible person. That lifetime reserve is 60 days, with a daily coinsurance fee of $476 (in 2006) (Centers for Medicare and Medicaid Services, 2005). The services provided by the hospital are those usually included within a hospital's per diem charges, but do not include the services of the anesthesiologist, pathologist, and radiologist. These services are charged separately by the doctors and are considered a Part B expense.

When patients have been hospitalized for at least 3 days and are found to be in need of treatment that cannot be provided in the home, but do not require hospital care, they may receive care in an extended care facility (ECF). These facilities are high-quality nursing homes that must be closely related to or have working agreements with a hospital and must be able to provide the kind of care the patient needs. Without additional charge, patients may receive up to 20 days of care in an ECF. An additional 80 days of care will be provided upon payment of a daily fee of $119 (in 2006) (Centers for Medicare and Medicaid Services, 2005). Few individuals will encounter these deductibles as the length of stay in hospitals has dropped drastically. In 2001, the median length of hospital stays for individuals enrolled in the Medicare program was between 5 and 6 days (Centers for Medicare and Medicaid Services, 2003). The service of an extended care facility shortens the length of stay of patients in hospitals; it is not intended to be long-term nursing home care. Indeed, the Medicare program as a whole does not respond to the need for long-term care.

If needed, home health care is available, with no ceiling on days and at no additional charge. Home health care must be medically ordered and must be of a medical nature, not homemaker service. The daily skilled care must be for a relatively short period of time or be seen as having an end within a predicted period. Medicare will reimburse hospices for the care they provide individuals with a terminal diagnosis of 6 months or less of life expectancy. The beneficiary may reside in a hospice for two 90-day periods and one subsequent 30-day period.

Part B

Part B of Medicare is called Supplemental Medical Insurance. As mentioned earlier, Medicare-eligible persons do not automatically participate in Part B. They agree to this insurance and pay $88.50 per month (in 2006) or accept that deduction being made from their Social Security checks (Centers for Medicare and Medicaid Services, 2005).

Nearly everyone receiving Social Security belongs to Part B, which provides partial payment for physicians for medical services. There is an annual deductible amount which, in 2006, was $124 (Centers for Medicare and Medicaid Services, 2005). Expenditures for drugs, dental services, and the like are not included in Part B. Individuals who have joined Part B, have paid their deductible amount of medical expenses, and have maintained monthly payments into the Part B fund are required to pay 20% of the charges Medicare determines are reasonable for a particular service. This 20% limit, however, does not apply to outpatient hospital services. For these outpatient services, the Medicare patient must pay 20% of whatever the hospital charges, rather than 20% of the amount approved by Medicare.

Outpatient psychiatric care was formerly reimbursed at a 50% rate with a $1,100 limit. This limit has now been removed. Medicare also now covers flu shots and routine mammograms every 2 years for women over age 65; Pap smears; screening for colon cancer, prostate cancer, and osteoporosis; and education for diabetics on self-testing and preventive treatment.

Physicians can be paid by making a direct charge to the federal Medicare agency (Centers for Medicare and Medicaid Services, 2003) through a system of intermediaries set up to deal directly with doctors. If they follow this route, they will receive 80% of the fee set by the intermediary, following the rules and directives of the agency. These rules, reflecting the concern in the Congress over the rise in medical costs in general and physicians' charges specifically, are directed toward keeping the Medicare payment in the general range of average payments and not at the level of higher charges made by some doctors. The doctor must look to the patient for the remaining 20% of his or her charges. Physicians must now submit their bill to Medicare, regardless of whether they do or do not accept assignment.

In the past, the fee was based on "reasonable and customary charges" in the community. As of 1992, the rates are based on a fee schedule developed through the Department of Health and Human Services. The fee schedule covers 7,000 services, and reimbursement is based on "value units" assigned to each procedure or medical service. These value units take into account the doctor's time, overhead, and risk of malpractice suit, and are then multiplied by a conversion factor in dollars. The resulting amount will be the Medicare approved rate. The importance of Medicare to the American health system can be illustrated with a few statistics: In 2004, 39 million older individuals were receiving Medicare benefits (Centers for Medicare and Medicaid Services, 2003). The estimated average annual benefit per person in 2004 was $6,800.

Medicare has encouraged older persons to join Health Maintenance Organizations (HMOs) that provide a wide range of care to their members on a prepayment basis. Under the Tax Equity and Fiscal Responsibility Act of 1982, older individuals who join HMOs continue to pay their Medicare Part B payments, and the HMO receives payment from the federal government for each member equivalent to 95% of the average Medicare costs in that state. The HMO must provide a range of services equivalent to that provided by Medicare. By 2003, 4.6 million Medicare beneficiaries had enrolled in these Medicare Advantage plans. One of the attractions of HMOs has been that they cover many costs not covered by Medicare, particularly those of prescription drugs and eyeglasses. After the initial large enrollment of seniors in HMOs, many plans dropped their coverage for the older persons. HMOs argued that the payments to provide for older persons were inadequate. These payments have now been raised and are often more than the payments provided through the traditional Medicare program (Pear, 2004). In 2004, 11.5% of Medicare beneficiaries were enrolled in HMOs and other private health care organizations (Pear, 2004).

The federal government has also experimented with Social HMOs (S/HMO), which provide additional social services to older recipients. The S/HMO experiment began in 1985 with an emphasis on case management. This model was found to be ineffective because of problems in coordination between case managers and care providers, particularly physicians. In 1996, a second model was initiated with an emphasis on assessment, geriatric care, and case management. S/HMOs provided for expanded Medicare reimbursement including prescription drugs and eyeglasses, personal care, and homemaker services. To cover these additional costs, S/HMO plans received 5.3% more than other HMOs that enroll

Medicare beneficiaries (Medicare +Choice plans). By 2003, 115,000 individuals were enrolled in four S/HMO plans (Medicare Payment Advisory Commission, 2003). Unfortunately, evaluations of the S/HMO experiment have not been positive. Enrollees were not more satisfied with the S/HMO services than those enrolled in Medicare +Choice plans. Most importantly, the S/HMO model did not produce consistent positive effects on the health or functional status of participants and did not consistently reduce the rate of hospitalization. Any reduction in the rates of hospitalization was balanced by a higher rate of skilled nursing home use than among Medicare +Choice enrollees. As a result of these evaluations, the Medicare Payment Advisory Commission unanimously recommended dismantling of the experiment and conversion of the S/HMO plans to the renamed Medicare Advantage plans (Medicare Payment Advisory Commission, 2003).

There have been two major gaps in Medicare funding: nursing home care and coverage for prescription drugs. Medicare funding for nursing home care is very limited. Long-term care is not included under Medicare because of its high cost and because it is a combination of both medical and domiciliary costs.

Coverage of prescription drugs began in 2006. Medicare beneficiaries pay a premium of approximately $30 per month for this coverage and the first $250 of the cost of their prescriptions. After the initial $250, Medicare reimburses the individual for 75% of the cost of prescriptions up to a total of $2,250. No more Medicare coverage is available until the cost of the prescriptions reaches $5,100 in that year, an expense for the older person of $3,600. Above $5,100, Medicare reimburses the individual for 95% of the cost. A "doughnut" approach appears to have been adopted because it would keep the total costs of this program down by not covering the costs between $2,250 and $5,100 but would provide more complete coverage for older persons with very heavy drug expenditures (over $5,100). It is likely that this approach and the figures used as cut-off points at each level will be altered in future years.

The prescription drug plans will be implemented through private insurers. By the end of September 2005, 10 national insurers had approved plans for offering Medicare prescription benefits. In larger states it was expected that beneficiaries would be able to choose from 20 different plans. Some of the plans may have a premium of only $20 per month but with expected higher out-of-pocket costs. In Oregon, 45 plans with premiums ranging from $7 to $65 were being offered at the end of 2005 (Pear, 2005b). Besides differences in premiums and deductibles, the plans will differ in their "formularies"—the drugs they will cover through their plan and the costs of the drugs. The law forbids Medicare from negotiating with the insurers on the costs of the drugs. Consumer advocates were concerned that the number of different insurers sending mailings and advertising on radio and television about their plans might confuse Medicare beneficiaries trying to decide which plan to join (Richwine, 2005).

Medicaid

This program, known officially as Medical Assistance, is much more complicated than Medicare. This is because Medicaid is a grant-in-aid to the states, requires state funding, and has a large element of state control. The federal law offers states the choice of whether they wish to have a Medicaid program and a variety of options on the breadth of eligibility, services covered, and fees to be paid. The result is considerable variation in the kinds of programs that have evolved in the states.

States must determine whether their Medicaid program is to be available only to people who receive payments from welfare programs, or whether the program will also include some of the medically needy. The welfare groups are those recipients of Temporary Aid to Needy Families (TANF) and SSI. With the inauguration of SSI in 1975, states were given a further option of excluding or including persons eligible under the expanded SSI program. The "medically needy" are those people who would qualify for the payment programs because of their high medical bills but whose incomes exceed the stated limits for eligibility. This distinction explains the large number of medically needy people who are not included in the Medicaid program. Among the excluded groups are those below the age of 65 who are not disabled. Those over age 65 would qualify for SSI, as would those under age 65 who are disabled. Another example is the intact family in which the father is employed but earns very little. As this family is not eligible for TANF, it is also not eligible for Medicaid.

About half of the states include some medically needy. In each of these states, a decision had to be made concerning the income level to be regarded as qualifying. Although federal law prevents states from being too liberal in making this decision, most states that include the medically needy have eligibility points below the federal maximum.

States must use Medicaid funds to pay for all Medicare premiums, co-payments, and deductibles for Medicare beneficiaries who are below the poverty line and have less than $4,000 in liquid assets. The Qualified Medicare Beneficiary (QMB) program has three levels. For the regular QMB individual, the program pays for the Medicare premiums, deductibles, and coinsurance. For the individual with slightly higher income (between 100% and 120% of the federal poverty level), the QMB program pays the cost of the Part B premium. The QMB program will also pay the costs of the premium for a limited number of individuals whose income level is between 120% and 135% of the federal poverty level (New York

State, Office for the Aging, 2004a). In 2002, 11% of enrollees in Part B of Medicare were part of this program (Centers for Medicare and Medicaid Services, 2003).

The federal law sets up the classifications of services that states must or can offer to pay for through Medicaid. States must offer some institutional and some noninstitutional services. In addition, states must offer:

- Inpatient hospital services
- Outpatient hospital services and other X-ray and laboratory services
- Skilled nursing home services for adults
- Early periodic screening services for children
- Physicians' services in the home, office, or hospital

For the medically needy, the states may offer a smaller range of services. In addition to those required services, there is a long list of other optional services, which includes drugs, home health care, dental services, and the like. A major optional service that the states may offer is intermediate care facility (ICF) care. An ICF provides services that range somewhere between those of a domiciliary facility and a nursing home. This obviously includes many nursing homes that offer only minimal services and often charge fees that the state Medicaid agency will pay. The federal share of Medicaid costs ranges from 50%, in states with per capita income equal to or greater than the national average, to 83%, for the state with the lowest per capita income in the United States.

By far the largest sums expended by the states for Medicaid are for hospitals, skilled nursing homes, and ICFs. Medicaid is the major source of public funds for long-term care. Inasmuch as all Medicare institutional services have time limits and the institutional services under Medicaid generally do not, many older persons find themselves receiving care in various kinds of nursing homes that are Medicaid-eligible. Federal law prohibits states from requiring that children be responsible for supporting parents. Even if older persons have resources in their own names, months of care in a nursing home will exhaust them. Thus, when the resources of the older persons diminish to the eligibility level for such resources as set by the state, they then become eligible for Medicaid.

Once a Medicaid recipient is institutionalized, states can place a lien on property to recover their Medicaid expenses, but not on the home of a spouse, children under the age of 21, or a blind or disabled child of any age. In addition, a lien cannot be placed on property where a brother or sister of the Medicaid recipient has equity if this sibling lived for at least 1 year in the home before the individual was institutionalized.

The Medicaid program has been engulfed in the rapidly rising cost of medical care. States have taken some steps to protect themselves, but even these measures have not been sufficiently effective to prevent the costs from becoming burdensome. In response to this, states have tended to trim services as best they can and have attempted to keep fees that they pay from rising too rapidly. The consequence is that many medical practitioners have refused to treat Medicaid patients. To some observers, the only answer to this problem of providing medical care for low-income people is national health insurance. To some degree, all national decisions around Medicaid have been regarded as temporary, made in the belief that national health insurance will surely come to be and will help solve the problems. Even as proposals continue, the prospects of such a national health plan still seem to be far in the future.

Private Health Insurance

A major force for paying medical costs in the United States is private health insurance. Public policy has supported the notion of a strong private sector for paying for medical care. Medical practitioners have encouraged it, industry has looked to the private sector to provide help to employees with their medical bills, and tax laws have encouraged the development of private health insurance plans.

Significant as private health insurance is, its impact is much less on the aged than on younger workers. Because so few of the aged are employed, they tend to have less private health insurance than do younger people. With the advent of Medicare in 1965, the private health insurance industry was pleased to assume a smaller role for the aged, for obvious reasons. There is great risk that the aged will become ill and will need costly medical services. Private insurance provides policies that supplement Medicare ("Medigap"). These policies pay for some of the deductibles and coinsurance charges and may provide payment for some additional hospital days, but they rarely cover long-term care. Thus, even the combination of Medicare and supplemental private health insurance does not provide the aged with full coverage. Long-term care insurance (discussed in Chapter 15) is becoming increasingly common among more affluent older persons.

Federal legislation now forbids the sale of duplicate policies and requires the salesperson to inquire whether the older person already has any medical policies. Salespeople must also list on the insurance application any other health insurance policies they have already sold to the older person, and the policies must return to the consumer at least 65% of what they bring in to the company.

Regulations adopted by the National Association of Insurance Commissioners now help to standardize Medigap policies. Under these regulations, 10 plans are offered. The basic plan offers "core" services.

These services include the coinsurance for Medicare Part A, 365 days of hospital coverage after Medicare benefits end, the 20% of doctors' fees not covered by Medicare, and the first three pints of blood a patient needs each year. The more extensive plans cover a variety of options including coverage during foreign travel, home care, preventive care, and prescription drugs. Consumers are thus able to make comparisons of the costs of each of these plans as offered by different insurers (Crenshaw, 1991). Unfortunately, increases in health care costs and utilization by older people have resulted in dramatic increases in Medigap premiums. In one area, a plan that covers 100% of all Medicare Part B costs and 50% of prescription drug costs up to $3,000 per year required a payment of $250 per month (New York State, Office for the Aging, 2004b).

Health insurance for older persons has become a complex, widely debated aspect of the American social welfare system. Clearly the existence of Medicare and other programs has provided a level of health care for older people that would formerly not have been possible. Despite the existence of all of these programs, however, the out-of-pocket medical expenses for older persons continue to be high. In 2003, older persons living outside of institutions such as nursing homes spent an average of $3,455 on their health care. This figure accounted for 22% of their income. Almost a quarter of the health care expenses of older persons were accounted for by payments for prescription drugs (Caplan & Brangan, 2004).

REFERENCES

Caplan, C., & Brangan, N. (2004). *Out-of-pocket spending on health care by Medicare beneficiaries age 65 and older in 2003*. Washington, DC: AARP Public Policy Institute.

Centers for Medicare and Medicaid Services. (2003). *Medicare state buy-ins for Supplemental Medical Insurance*. Retrieved October 23, 2004, from http://www.cms.hhs.gov/researchers/pubs/datacompendium/2003/03pg33.xls

Centers for Medicare and Medicaid Services. (2005). *Medicare premiums and coinsurance rates for 2006*. Retrieved October 17, 2005, from http://medicare.questions.gov

Crenshaw, A. (1991, October 16). Relief for Medigap confusion. *Washington Post*, Family and Retirement Section, p. 6.

Federal Hospital Insurance Trust Fund. (1998). *Annual report*. Retrieved December 20, 2004, from http://http://medicare.commission.gov/medicare/factpage4.html

Medicare Payment Advisory Commission. (2003). *Report to the Congress: Social Health Maintenance Organization (S/HMO): Recommendations for the future of the demonstration*. Retrieved from http://www.medpac.gov/publications/congressional-report/Auh03_SHMO-SHMO%20Report.pdf

National Center for Health Statistics. (1991). *1989 summary: National Hospital Discharge Survey.* Hyattsville, MD: Author.

New York State, Office for the Aging. (2004a). *Help for the low income Medicare beneficiaries.* Retrieved October 23, 2004, from http://hiicap.state.ny.us/medicare/lowincome.htm

New York State, Office for the Aging. (2004b). *Monthly premiums for Medigap plans.* Retrieved October 23, 2004, from http://hiicap.state.ny.us/mgap/mgap05a.htm

Pear, R. (2004, September 17). Private plans costing more for Medicare. *New York Times,* pp. 17, A12.

Pear, R. (2005a, January 11). Nation's health spending slows, but it still hits a record. *New York Times,* p. A14.

Pear, R. (2005b, October 1). Drug plans in Medicare are starting marketing. *New York Times,* p. A8.

Richwine, L. (2005). Ten firms to offer Medicare drug plans nationally. Retrieved September 29, 2005, from http://news.yahoo.com/s/nm/20050923/hl_nm/medicare_dc

Rosenbaum, D. (2005, March 24). Medicare outlook called direr than Social Security's. *New York Times,* p. A15.

U.S. House of Representatives, Committee on Ways and Means. (1986). *Background material and data on programs within the jurisdiction of the Committee on Ways and Means.* Washington, DC: U.S. Government Printing Office.

PART III

Programs for the Aged

Existing programs and services can be classified according to the dependence of the individuals assisted. Programs and services can also be classified as home help, medical, financial, assessment, referral, social-recreational, and transportation.

Many of the programs and services included in this list have common elements. Adult day care centers and multipurpose senior centers utilize transportation and have major social components. Although this volume often discusses providing "services" or "serving" the elderly, the attempt is to differentiate between programs and services, terms often used synonymously. As defined, "programs" contain individual elements; "services" include many of these same elements combined under a larger umbrella. These programs and services are discussed as they are most commonly organized, but the existence of state-by-state variations means that descriptions of a program or service may be more applicable to one area than another.

In this part the focus is on individual programs vital to the well-being of the elderly: information and assistance, health and mental health programs, transportation, crime prevention and legal assistance programs, employment, volunteer programs, educational programs, and nutrition programs.

CHAPTER FIVE

Information and Assistance

GOALS

Creating an extensive network of services has no benefits for older persons unless they are informed about the availability of these services and how to make use of them. Information and assistance programs are thus a natural outgrowth of the tremendous increase in public and private programs for the elderly. The size of the agencies giving services, the size of the population being served in a given geographic area, and the number of different services available determine the need for an information exchange system that can identify appropriate services.

For the population at large, including the elderly, information and assistance is a social service in its own right: an activity by which a person in need is made aware of, and connected to, a service or resource that can meet the need. However, the simple concept of establishing a link between need and resource becomes complex as one takes a closer look.

The functions of information and assistance for the elderly are essentially the same as those for the general population, except for the focus on the specific needs of the elderly: (1) the assemblage and provision of information to link older persons with the services designed to help them meet their particular problems, and (2) the collection and reporting of information about the needs of older people and the adequacy of resources available to them. Information and assistance systems link individuals to services and services to each other. The OAA also emphasizes the need for follow-up to ensure that individuals receive the services they need.

HISTORY

Information and assistance programs began in the 1960s when monies were increasing for social programs. Some large federal and state agencies offered information and referral to the public in response to an expressed need. Information was provided in booklets and over the telephone as the need arose.

Official federal interest in information and assistance began in 1971, with the passage of legislation authorizing the Social Security Administration to provide information to wage earners who would soon be retiring. In 1973, under the Comprehensive Service Amendments to the Older Americans Act (OAA), priority was given to the development of information and assistance programs for the elderly. Similarly, the information and assistance needs of the general welfare population, including the elderly, were addressed under the 1974/1975 Title XX social services regulations, which designated these as optional services that states could elect to provide. However, information and assistance services were mandatory for SSI recipients. Title II of the Community Services Act of 1974 provided for urban and rural community action programs. Under a special section for Senior Opportunities and Services, provisions were made for information and assistance programs, which could also be operated under the National Health Planning and Resources Development Act of 1974 and the Community Mental Health Centers Amendments of 1975. In addition, a series of interagency agreements have been developed at the federal level to promote coordination of information and assistance services through joint efforts at the federal, state, and local levels.

Information and assistance have grown in importance with each reauthorization of the Older Americans Act. The 1992 amendments required the AoA Commissioner to establish information and assistance as a priority service. In Title III, plans submitted by an Area Agency on Aging must not only discuss the establishment of information and assistance programs, but must also emphasize the linkage of isolated elderly suffering from Alzheimer's disease or related disorders to programs and services. Many of the components of Title VII involve information and assistance. A major example is the Outreach, Counseling, and Assistance Program.

OPERATION AND FUNCTIONS

A truly productive information and assistance system not only will be able to generate and respond to questions of need but will also test the degree to which the belief that adequate services exist is based on fact. Information and assistance systems thus have the potential for generating beneficial changes in the service system. An effective information and assistance system cannot work outside the service system. Its success is dependent, at least in part, on the extent and quality of the service system to which it refers.

An information and assistance system provides information about the service system and generates information through frequent contact with the services available. Information and assistance programs can be helpful to clients only if the service agencies have a clear understanding of what they are actually providing. Because the information given by agencies is not always an accurate portrayal of what is available, some information and assistance programs use client-supplied data to revise their descriptions. In addition, once the information about the agencies has been stored, it can be used as important data for planning and development purposes. Follow-up on clients receiving information from the information and assistance program can indicate the effectiveness of the service response.

ORGANIZATION

Scope

The diversity of information and assistance programs almost matches the number of information and assistance services available throughout the country, a number difficult to quantify because information sharing takes many forms. In order to identify a minimum requirement for an adequate information and assistance program, the federal Administration on Aging prepared policy guidelines to state agencies administering plans under the provisions of the OAA. Issued in August 1974, these guidelines also discuss long-range goals for the development of comprehensive information and assistance programs.

The nine service components were designed to build uniformity and comprehensiveness into the information and assistance programs and to provide some measure of adequacy. The service components emphasized:

1. having an adequate facility to serve those seeking information,
2. making continuously updated resource files available to agencies needing service information,
3. making the service easily available to older persons,
4. providing outreach to those not familiar with using such a service,
5. following up on referrals, and
6. providing transportation when necessary to help the older person reach a service identified through information and assistance.

The individual who calls or walks into an information and assistance service is assured of anonymity, and usually no names are recorded on data forms. A casework approach is often utilized, in which the information and assistance worker explores the individual's problem and the alternative services available. As needed, the older person is referred to a specific service.

Schmandt, Bach, and Radin (1979) attempted to bring some clarity to the wide range of efforts that fall under the information and assistance label. Their attempt again indicated the complexity of the seemingly simple function of information and assistance. An information and assistance program may define its clientele on the basis of age, income, or specific problems. The program may confine itself to telephone assistance or move into extensive outreach, including contact with individuals in their own homes. Limited research on the needs of the population within the community may also be undertaken. Within a defined city or metropolitan area, the agency offering the information and assistance program may adopt a posture that emphasizes a personal type of relationship with clients, or, alternatively, a relatively impersonal and highly professional one.

One of the difficulties in identifying and maintaining a minimum standard for information and assistance programs is the pressure to have these programs reflect the style, service system, and needs of the locale in which they are located. Schmandt and colleagues (1979) argued for both the standardized and localized programs, including a centralized telephone center as well as decentralized walk-in centers in local neighborhoods. A two-part system of this type can effectively respond to the multifaceted needs of a variety of clients in the local community.

A range of institutions are involved in the planning and delivery of information and assistance programs. As indicated earlier, at the federal level, information and assistance responsibilities for the elderly are shared by a number of agencies. State and county social service departments represent a second layer of organizations responsible for information and assistance functions. At the community level, a variety of public and private organizations dispense information and assistance, generally to populations that include the elderly as well as other groups.

Types of Programs Available

The types of information generation, storage, and retrieval systems used are essential to determining the success of information and assistance. If local structures and community needs are taken into consideration when choosing a type of system, the system has a greater chance of success. A local walk-in information and assistance program has different information needs than a program that serves a large region and supplies data for planning. The service that can clarify its informational goals can be more effectively evaluated.

It has been suggested that the availability of late-hour and toll-free telephone lines would increase the success of information and assistance efforts. In 1990 the Administration on Aging awarded a grant to the National Association of Area Agencies on Aging to develop a toll-free 800 number that would refer callers to services in their area. The ElderCare Locator, now sponsored by the National Association of Area Agencies on Aging and the National Association of State Units on Aging, provides information on current services in an area, the location of the services, and the type of services being offered. It is also available online to individuals with access to the Internet.

The basic purpose of information and assistance programs is to provide information to individuals. The ability of these services to fulfill this function is difficult to evaluate from the perspective of users because "many users do not conceptually separate the information and referral service from the actual service provider" (Burkhardt, 1979, p. 30). Individuals tend to call an information and assistance service when faced with an immediate problem. In the vast majority of cases, they are referred to an agency or specialized service for assistance. Thus clients' perceptions of the effectiveness of information and assistance may be intertwined with how well they felt the agency to which they were referred dealt with their needs.

If information and assistance programs provide links to appropriate services they can increase the probability that clients will receive the services they need. In this effort information and assistance programs can undertake a number of steps:

- Refer a client directly to one or more agencies
- Arrange for transportation or escort to ensure that the client can reach the referred service
- Go to the client's home to provide direct assistance
- Call the service provider directly, giving information about the client, and then tell the client that the necessary contact has been made

One of the big problems of information and assistance programs, as with any program available to the elderly, is accessibility to anyone who needs the service. The information and assistance program has the potential of being the most widely available of any service for the elderly because it is relatively inexpensive and equally accessible to everyone. However, despite this relative accessibility, information and assistance programs are used by a disproportionate number of people who are already connected into the system in some way. The lack of awareness about many programs is probably most acute among lower-income minority elderly. A study of reservation-based, urban and rural Native American elderly in Michigan indicated that only 25% of these older persons knew about all of the services available to them (Chapleski, Gelfand, & Pugh, 1997). Resource centers such as the National Resource Center on Native American Aging at the University of North Dakota are attempting to provide information on aging programs and services to Native American communities around the country (National Resource Center on Native American Aging, n.d.). Unfortunately, direct outreach is expensive, and many such programs do not have adequate funds. When funds are limited, extensive use of the media appears the best way to reach isolated elderly populations. It is thus likely that most information and assistance services will not undertake the wide range of follow-up and client advocacy functions that are possible for their programs.

Several programs have been established in recent years to decrease the number of steps required before an individual obtains appropriate assistance from a variety of organizations. These programs utilize information and assistance programs as their base, but go further in their assistance. In Maryland, the Senior Care program helps to ensure some coordination among the agencies that provide services. An interagency committee in each of Maryland's 24 jurisdictions helps to ensure that older persons are having all of their health and social services needs met. In 1999, 2,500 people received services through this program (Maryland Department of Aging, 1999).

Many states have also developed local senior information and assistance centers that are housed in senior centers and other organizational settings. These centers provide information and assistance including information on Social Security, housing, income/financial assistance, health care, transportation, legal assistance, employment, nutrition/food support, home repair, and leisure activities. This material is also usually available on the state's Internet sites.

With the inclusion of the National Family Caregiver Support Program in the 2000 OAA amendments, an increasing number of information and assistance programs have been developed for caregivers of older individuals. Assisted by funding from AoA, the program provided assistance to more than 325,000 caregivers by 2002. In addition to information and assistance, counseling, respite, and supplemental services have been provided (Administration on Aging, 2002). AoA and state Web sites now provide substantial information to caregivers about available services in their area. In Illinois, Caregiver Resource Centers have been placed in local senior centers and other settings around the states. AoA is also supporting innovative efforts that attempt to further caregiving efforts through local corporations and health organizations.

Active older adults also need information about their living options. Since 1998 New Jersey has offered a Community Choice program in which registered nurses and social workers provide information for older individuals who have been discharged from a hospital or nursing home. The program helps them understand and choose between returning to their own homes or other options such as board and care homes or assisted living (Community Choice, 2004).

Funding

Funding for information and assistance programs comes from a variety of federal, state, local, and private sources, although state and area agencies contribute a larger percentage of funds than do other types of contributors. Major federal resources available include the Administration on Aging or the Community Services block grant. A variety of other funding sources are used for information and assistance programs. These range from monies provided by nonprofit community groups such as the United Way to local foundations and corporations and income generated by the programs themselves through sales of brochures, directories, and planning information.

IMPORTANCE

Information and assistance programs can be the link between the individual needing some type of service that can best meet that person's needs and relevant programs. According to the National Council on the Aging (1982), the effective information and assistance system must be:

- confidential
- accessible to all older persons
- sensitive to feelings and problems of older persons
- friendly to older clients
- reliable and accurate in the information it provides
- accountable and responsive to older persons and families
- neutral and nonpartisan in its referrals
- broad in the range of information it provides

Many older people are unaware of the kinds of services available and how they can be found and, in many cases, are approaching the thought of professional assistance for the first time in their adult lives. A well-implemented information and assistance program can make older people aware of services, help them formulate their problem in the context of available services, and assist them in actually making the contact with the appropriate service. Organizing the maze of possible service systems, regulations, and eligibility requirements into a package of information, the information and assistance program is essential for responsive service delivery to the elderly, regardless of the size of the community. Just as information and assistance cannot be effective without a good service delivery system, service delivery systems cannot be effective without an efficient information and assistance program: one that reaches to everyone in need of problem solving.

REFERENCES

Administration on Aging. (2002). *2002 annual report: What we do makes a difference*. U.S. Department of Health and Human Services, Administration on Aging. Retrieved July 23, 2004, from http://www.aoa.gov

Burkhardt, J. (1979). Evaluating information and referral services. *Gerontologist, 19*, 28–33.

Chapleski, E., Gelfand, D., & Pugh, K. (1997). Great Lakes American Indian elders and service utilization: Does residence matter? *Journal of Applied Gerontology, 16*, 333–354.

Community Choice. (2004). Trenton, NJ: New Jersey Department of Health and Senior Services.

Maryland Department of Aging. (1999). *Consumer satisfaction and effect of the Senior Care system in Maryland*. Retrieved July 27, 2004, from http://www.mdoa.state.md.us/services/SCsurvey.pdf

National Council on the Aging. (1982). *Comprehensive service delivery through senior centers and other community focal points: A resource manual*. Washington, DC: Author.

National Resource Center on Native American Aging. (n.d.). Retrieved October 10, 2005, from http://www.med.und.nodak.edu/depts/rural//nrcnaa/overview/index.html

Schmandt, J., Bach, V., & Radin, B. (1979). Information and referral services for the elderly welfare recipients. *Gerontologist, 19*, 21–27.

CHAPTER SIX

Health and Mental Health

As noted in Chapter 1, older persons often suffer from a variety of chronic illnesses. The older adult does not suffer from the common cold as much as arthritis, the effects of strokes, and vision and hearing problems. Medical care for a population with these types of problems must stress not only efforts to cure, but treatment that allows the individual to adjust to living with a condition that may vary in intensity but will always be present.

Attempts to provide medical care for the elderly have met a variety of roadblocks including: (1) the lack of interest by physicians in treating individuals whose conditions are not "curable," (2) the high costs of medical care, and (3) the inaccessibility of medical treatment. These problems are also endemic in mental health treatment of the elderly.

Medicare and Medicaid have helped to reduce the cost of medical care for many older adults, although the out-of-pocket share of medical expenses incurred by the elderly has been increasing consistently. Specialized transportation programs for older adults have also targeted medical appointments as a top priority. A major problem that remains to be addressed is the recruitment and training of professionals and paraprofessionals dedicated to providing medical care for seniors. Until the mid-1970s, there was little emphasis on geriatrics in American schools of medicine. The curriculum in most medical schools has only recently begun to include any appreciable content on the aging process.

Even if physicians show increased interest in treating the elderly, hospitals are oriented toward acute illnesses, and individuals who remain hospitalized for an extended length of time run up enormous bills. The alternative to acute care hospitals—a long stay in a nursing home—has not been attractive to the elderly or their families.

The introduction of in-home services, adult day care centers, and assisted living has made care outside of hospitals and nursing homes

possible. The majority of health care programs serving the elderly are
part of the extensive range of home care services that are becoming avai -
able. In this chapter we will examine health care programs available
through clinics, hospitals, and non-home care agencies.

With the elderly spending substantial amounts of money for health
care, the question has arisen as to whether separate services should be developed that are oriented to older adults. Separate services may require
duplication of facilities and equipment. Older individuals who feel stigmatized by attending special clinics may avoid these facilities.
Alternatively, whereas encouraging the elderly to utilize existing services
may avoid major capital outlays, older patients at large clinics often receive less attention from health professionals who are attracted to
younger, more "curable" clients. With younger clients being generally
more assertive about the health care to which they feel entitled, the net result is that the elderly are often relegated to long waits and poor care.

HEALTH CARE PROGRAMS

Geriatric Clinics

A geriatric health clinic in a medical center is a compromise service delivery system that avoids setting up new facilities, but guarantees the
elderly that their medical needs will receive attention. At Syracuse
University, a geriatric clinic was integrated with other community health
facilities. The clinic planners hoped that this integration would help to
avoid ostracization of the elderly. Patients were assisted in establishing a
relationship with a physician, but the clinic also maintained a referral
service for specialized medical problems not treatable at the clinic
(Syracuse University School of Social Work, 1971). Geriatric clinics are
now common at many medical centers. An example is the Geriatric
Assessment Clinic operated by the Department of Family Medicine at the
University of Iowa. This multidisciplinary program is staffed by physicians, social workers, pharmacists, and chaplains and provides an extensive assessment of the behavioral and physical needs of an older patient.
As efforts have increased to reach many diverse populations of older people, interdisciplinary health teams have become aware of their need for a
greater understanding of the many cultural groups they are serving. The
result is more extensive training to ensure that practitioners are "culturally
competent." Cultural competence is a major component of the University
of Pennsylvania Interdisciplinary Geriatric Fellowship Program.

Health screening programs are now common at senior centers, and
many are held in May during Older Americans Month. The Waxter

Senior Center in Baltimore has an affiliation with the University of Maryland Department of Internal Medicine. The department operates a health clinic at the senior center. St. Patrick's Senior Center in Detroit has a health clinic staffed by physicians and nurses from the Detroit Medical Center. In some areas, mobile vans are utilized for health screening programs.

The Program for All-Inclusive Care for Elders (PACE) is one of the most ambitious efforts to provide interdisciplinary health care for older adults. Begun by San Francisco's On Lok Senior Center in 1979, PACE now has 35 sites that target the frail elderly who are eligible for nursing homes. The services at the sites range from social and medical services, home care, transportation, meals, and personal counseling. In 2002, 8,350 individuals were served by PACE programs (Kornblatt, Cheng, & Chan, 2002). The typical PACE client is an 80-year-old woman, with 7.9 medical conditions and problems in carrying out three of the Activities of Daily Living. Although 40% of PACE clients evidence some degree of dementia, 90% can still live in the community (PACE, 2004).

Health Promotion

Local primary prevention programs have been built around educational programs informing the elderly about nutrition, care of chronic illnesses, correct drug usage, and a variety of other medical issues. These educational programs have been run at senior centers, nutrition sites, and adult day care centers. Short television and radio announcements have also been utilized in efforts to alert the elderly to potential health problems and appropriate treatment. Health fairs have been inaugurated in many localities. These one-day fairs provide information on a variety of health conditions and programs and offer basic screening of blood pressure, vision, and hearing.

Exercise Programs

In recent years, it has become evident that regular exercise is an important element of illness prevention for individuals of all ages. Increasing numbers of senior centers, as well as day care programs, are offering exercise classes and activities for their clients. One innovative intergenerational effort is the Adult Health Development Clinic at the University of Maryland. The clinic meets on Saturdays. Over the course of 11 weeks, 60–120 students work with the older participants and assist in morning exercises and physical activities. The relationships developed through this one-to-one contact often extend into close friendships between students and older persons (Adult Health and Development Program, 2004).

Dental Care

Dental problems increase with age. An estimated 70% of individuals over the age of 65 have had tooth pain in the last 6 months (Vargas, Kramarow, & Yellowitz, 2001). In addition, many drugs that older people take for a variety of health problems produce dry mouth. The reduction in saliva increases the risk for oral disease (National Institute of Dental and Craniofacial Research, 2000).

Older persons who do not have dental insurance often omit regular dental checkups. Dental care is not reimbursed through Medicare, and most states do not cover it through Medicaid. The net effect of this lack of care is very negative. In 1993, one-third of non-institutionalized older persons had none of their regular teeth. This figure is even higher among nursing home residents because of the lack of adequate dental programs in these facilities.

Efforts are being fostered to make regular dental care affordable for older adults. In some states, dental societies are beginning to work with senior centers and Area Agencies on Aging to offer dental care to elderly clients at reduced rates. This reduced-rate dental care may be provided at dentists' offices, but some senior centers are also incorporating dental suites into their facilities. These facilities also serve as training sites for dental students.

Drugs

As major consumers of both prescription and over-the-counter drugs, the elderly are faced with the problems of absorbing the enormous costs of these medications, even when assisted by Medicare and Medicaid.

The shift in many states to utilization of generic rather than brand-name drugs helps to lower costs for drugs whose patent years have expired. Beginning in 1958, AARP has operated direct-mail pharmacies for its members. Many older persons have explored the cost savings resulting from ordering their medications online. For those Americans living close to Canada, a trip across the border to fill their prescriptions at Canadian pharmacies has resulted in significant savings. As a result of continued discussion of the high costs of prescriptions, Congress responded in 2003 with passage of the Medicare prescription drug benefit. This was a first effort on the part of Congress to alleviate the burden faced by older persons requiring extensive numbers of medications.

Beyond providing drugs at lower costs, a number of programs are now directed to providing more consumer education about the potentials as well as the dangers of drugs. Pharmacies now distribute leaflets with prescriptions that provide details about correct usage of the drugs. In addition, pharmacists maintain personal profiles that keep an inventory of the drugs older consumers may be taking. This effort enables pharmacists to alert consumers when drugs, often prescribed by different doctors, may cause dangerous interactions. Programs to educate older persons about the interaction effects of drugs are also available at many senior centers.

All of these diverse efforts will need to be greatly expanded in the future if the requisite health care for the elderly is to be provided. As the numbers of older persons living in the community increases, a larger complement of health care programs will be needed to prevent and treat acute and chronic illnesses prevalent among older adults.

MENTAL HEALTH PROGRAMS

In the United States, mental hospitals have often functioned as quasi-homes for the aged. This approach changed with the onset of community mental health programs in the 1960s and the growing movement in the 1970s to "deinstitutionalize" patients. By the 1990s, the number of inpatients had dropped from a high of 559,000 in 1955 to fewer than 100,000 across the United States (Grob, 2000). In the late 1990s, older adults comprised only 7% of individuals receiving inpatient mental health services (American Association for Geriatric Psychiatry, 2004).

Community Mental Health

Community mental health programs took root in 1963 with the passage of the Community Mental Health Centers Act. The intention of the Act's supporters was to enlarge mental health expenditures at all levels and develop a network of community-based treatment facilities, which would be located in geographic areas that had a maximum population of 175,000. Each state, however, had to determine appropriate catchment area boundaries. In each catchment area an organization was to be designated as responsible for providing community mental health services.

As originally specified in 1963, the services included five major components. In 1975, this list was enlarged to a total of 12 different services:

1. Inpatient care
2. Outpatient care
3. Partial hospitalization (day care)
4. Emergency services
5. Consultation and education
6. Specialized services for children

7. Specialized services for the elderly
8. Screening of individuals considered for referral to a state menta hospital
9. Follow-up services for discharged inpatients
10. Transitional halfway houses for former mental patients
11. Programs for prevention and treatment of alcoholism if not already in existence in the catchment area
12. Programs for the prevention and treatment of drug addiction, if not already available in the catchment area.

Beginning in 1981, federal funds were awarded to states under a block grant program. The Mental Health Services Block Grant specified five required services: outpatient services, 24-hour-a-day emergency services, day treatment, screening of patients for state mental health facilities, and consultation and education.

Primary prevention, as embodied in the consultation and education programs, was one of the major assumptions of community mental health services. Treatments for individual mental health problems were supposed to be supplemented by primary prevention programs that located the sources of stress in the environment and worked with community groups to alleviate these negative influences. Primary prevention efforts focused on at-risk populations would include the elderly in many communities.

The OAA did not specifically recognize the importance of mental health services for older persons until 1987. In the amendments passed that year, the term "mental health" was added at many points where formerly only the term "health" had been used. Any mental health services provided with AAA funds were to be coordinated with community mental health center programs and those of other public and nonprofit agencies. Even with this emphasis older adults comprised only 6% of community mental health clients (Administration on Aging, 2001). The emphasis of these programs is on individuals with severe chronic mental illness. As a result, only four states have designated older people in general as a priority population for mental health services (Administration on Aging, 2001).

Mental Health Prevention Programs

Bereavement programs offered through many organizations, including hospices, help widows and widowers deal with mental health issues associated with loss of a spouse. Peer counseling has also been found to be effective in helping seniors deal with mental health concerns. Part of the growth of peer counseling programs can be explained by the belief that older people will more readily talk to their age peers than to younger cohorts. Peer counselors can also serve as positive role models for the individuals they counsel (Bratter & Freeman, 1990).

In Santa Monica, California, a peer counseling program was begun in 1977. By 1990, 208 counselors had been trained. Each counselor must volunteer for 8 hours per week for 1 year after training (Bratter, 1986). The model developed in Santa Monica has been adopted by many other cities. In San Francisco, the Senior Peer Counseling program of the Family Service Agency provides 2½-hour weekly training sessions over 7 weeks for volunteers. The trained volunteers are then matched with up to three other seniors with whom they work to deal with mental health concerns (Family Service Agency of San Francisco, 2004).

Deinstitutionalization

During the 1960s, mental hospitals were derided, not only for their effects on individuals and the lack of adequate treatment, but also for their supposedly high costs. Proponents of community-based programs argued that individuals could be treated outside the state mental hospital without creating an "institutional personality" and at a lower cost. Actual experiences have not always shown these cost claims to be true. Although state mental hospital costs are evident upon careful auditing, accounting for the costs of a community-based program is more difficult.

> Mrs. S. provides a good example. A woman in her early 70s, she had been in the state hospital for 20 years. Discharged under the new community approach of the 1960s, Mrs. S. has been living in an old hotel in a beachfront community in New York. Because of her lack of any other means of support, she receives financial aid from the state as well as casework services from the Department of Social Services. The mental health services she obtains are provided through the Department of Mental Hygiene. If any vocational training is included in the support she receives, it will be provided by the Department of Vocational Rehabilitation. Mrs. S. is thus receiving a variety of services, most of which are not provided under mental health auspices. These services are therefore not counted in the cost of the mental health programs.

Discharged mental patients living in old hotels and domiciliary facilities operated by state mental health departments continue to make headlines, as many communities protest these problems being "dumped" in their neighborhoods. As some communities pass zoning regulations, making it difficult to open new facilities, discharged mental patients become concentrated in areas such as Long Beach, New York; South Miami;

or parts of Chicago. Charges have been made that many of these group homes "warehouse" patients and provide inadequate standards. In 2004, a group home in New York City settled charges that its 24 schizophrenic residents had been illegally subjected to prostate surgery in a money-making scheme for the home's owners and two urologists. This same home had already been found to be in violation of many building codes including vermin infestation, soiled linen, damaged walls and ceilings, and the poor hygienic condition of the residents (Levy, 2004). Unfortunately, in cases such as this, state agencies delay closing a facility because they have little recourse to other, better facilities for the residents. Because of a lack of adequate facilities, many individuals with severe mental health problems have joined the ranks of the homeless, creating the unfortunate impression among many urban residents that all homeless individuals have mental problems.

Mental patients have also shown up in increasing numbers among prison populations. In 2000, it was estimated that 200,000 prison inmates were suffering from schizophrenia, manic depression, or major depression (Butterfield, 2000). The Los Angeles County jail had more than 1,500 inmates who were classified as severely mentally ill (Butterfield, 2000). One psychiatrist, Eugene Kunzman, noted that the current inmates of many prisons were the same types of patients he formerly worked with in state mental hospitals (Butterfield, 2000). Few jail systems, however, are able to adequately provide the mental health services needed by individuals with major mental health problems.

ELDERLY IN THE MENTAL HEALTH SYSTEM

There are now three major groups of elderly involved in the mental health system: (1) elderly who have been long-term residents of state hospitals and are attempting to live outside the controlled hospital environment, (2) elderly who have been utilizing mental health services for a period of time, and (3) elderly who begin to exhibit major mental health problems only as they become older. These problems may include depression, insomnia, hypochondria, paranoia, and organic brain disorders. We will examine the present condition of mental health services for former residents of state hospitals and for older persons exhibiting mental health problems often associated with aging.

Mental Health and Nursing Homes

Many nursing home residents have mental health problems, and the need for expanded mental health services in these settings has been evident for many years. In a 1976 report, Glasscote and colleagues summarized an investigation of the mental health needs and treatment of nursing home patients:

> Our sample of nursing facilities estimated that about three quarters of their patients are either formally diagnosed with a psychiatric disorder or are "de facto psychiatrically impaired"; if this figure can be projected to the 1,100,000 population of all nursing homes, then there are more than three quarters of a million nursing home patients with psychiatric disability, most of whom have had no contact at all with psychiatrists. [p. 71]

In 1999, the National Nursing Home Survey reported that 20% of the almost 1.5 million nursing home residents over the age of 65 in the United States had received mental health services 30 days before the survey. A significant percentage of the residents (16.5%) had a mental disorder as their primary diagnosis when admitted to the nursing home (Access to disability data, 2004). Katz (2003) estimated that 80% of nursing home residents had psychological problems, particularly depression.

In 1987, Congress required that applicants for nursing homes be screened for mental health problems. Screening may be partly responsible for the 108% increase between 1977 and 1987 in the number of nursing home residents diagnosed with a mental health disorder (Smyer, Shea, & Streit, 1994). Individuals who need treatment must be provided this treatment by a nursing home. Prior to passage of this legislation it is estimated that only 4.5% of nursing home residents were receiving mental health treatment, a figure much lower than any available estimates of need. Among those receiving treatment, the most common diagnosis was schizophrenia (Burns et al., 1993).

In Michigan, the Birchwood Nursing Center in Traverse City provides specialized mental health services for its residents (Michigan program links, 1990). Programs of this kind are not widespread in nursing homes. Special mental health treatment programs have been found in only 34 skilled nursing facilities, accounting for only 3,384 beds from the more than 1 million total (Stortz, 2003).

Elderly in Mental Health Centers

For the majority of the over-60 population, mental health services must be obtained from community mental health centers. As already shown, services to the elderly were a requirement for federally funded mental health centers. Despite this mandate of 1975, these centers have still not shown a major interest in providing extensive mental health services for older adults. For the majority of mental health professionals, the most desirable clients remain youthful, and successful individuals (Wei, Sambamoorthi, & Olfson, 2005). In contrast, the elderly are often perceived as depressed individuals whose problems are merely the products of getting old. Whereas the younger persons have an extensive future ahead of them, mental health professionals may view older persons as having their best years behind them, and thus as less deserving of attention.

Some members of the present generation of elderly may also fail to utilize mental health services because of their limited education and fluency in English. Other more complex reasons are that they may (1) not recognize some behaviors as mental health problems, (2) believe that many mental health problems are the responsibility of the family unless extremely serious (Fandetti & Gelfand, 1978), (3) stigmatize mental illness and be fearful of being labeled "crazy" if it becomes known that they are utilizing mental health services, (4) be unaware of the services available at mental health centers, or (5) have difficulty reaching mental health centers and clinics because of lack of transportation.

At present, the mental health needs of the elderly are much more extensive than the services provided. The prevalence of mental illness and emotional distress among older individuals is higher than among younger populations. The estimates are that 20% of the population over the age of 55 experience mental health problems. One significant behavioral indicator of these problems is that the suicide rate for older adults is higher than for any other age group. Among individuals over the age of 85 the suicide rate is twice the national average (American Association for Geriatric Psychiatry, 2004). Mental health problems may also be evident in community-based programs: 37% of clients in adult day centers in Seattle had significant mental health problems (Washington State, Mental Health Division, 2003).

SPECIALIZED AGING SERVICES

The switch in mental health funding from a "categorical" system to the block grant system removed specific requirements for mental health services for the elderly. Under the block grant system, decisions about specific priority groups for mental health services are now made at the state level.

Some AAAs have recognized the relationship between social and mental health services. In Washington, a service agreement between the Spokane Community Mental Health Center and the Eastern Washington Area Agency on Aging has been based on the assumption that "mental health needs of the elderly, especially frail, vulnerable, or moderately to severely dysfunctional cannot be separated from physical, social and economic needs" (Raschko, 1985, p. 461).

The Michigan Office of Services to the Aging and the state Department of Mental Health have implemented a program ("Building

Ties") through which participating counties designate a liaison person to help coordinate mental health services for older persons. In Indiana, a mental health center staff person is placed for a half day per week at a senior center, nutrition center, or public housing project. This staff person conducts educational programs, in-service training on mental health, group discussions, case and program consultation, as well as reduced-fee individual counseling (Michigan program, 1990).

The Psychogeriatric Assessment, Treatment, and Teaching program in Baltimore utilizes two nurses and two psychiatrists to conduct mental health outreach efforts in public housing with a large population of older residents. The residents are referred to the PATCH team by building management (Roca, Storer, Robbins, Tlasek, & Rabins, 1990). A follow-up study of PATCH found that 26 months after their referral to this program, older clients had significantly lower psychiatric symptoms than a control group (Rabins et al., 2000). In Seattle, the In-Home Mental Health Program offers mental health services to older clients in diverse settings such their own home, assisted living facilities, and nursing homes (Washington State, Mental Health Division, 2003).

In Florida, Jewish Family Services (JFS) of the Gulf Coast has implemented three major mental health programs for residents of the area. The Geriatric Residential Treatment System is a community-based residential treatment program. Begun in 1980, this program has served 2,000 individuals over the age of 50 through community residence, case management, and day treatment. At the Hacienda Home, 60 beds are available and an interdisciplinary team is available for assistance to individuals with severe mental problems. JFS also conducts an Alternative Family program that provides foster homes for 225 chronically ill individuals (Gulf Coast Jewish Family Services, 2004).

Funding

Mental health programs are often viewed as expensive. Unlike sufferers of many acute illnesses, individuals with mental health problems may embark on a long period of treatment, including therapists and expensive medication. As a result, many private insurance plans limit their mental health coverage. Even Part B of the Medicare program only reimburses mental health services at a 50% rate, compared to the 80% reimbursement for other health services. As already indicated, the movement of patients out of psychiatric hospitals was expected to result in cost savings but this has not been evident in many states. In addition, the stigmatization of mental health problems often makes it easier to cut funds for these programs than for other health endeavors.

Mental health funding has failed to keep up with the need to provide services. The federal Mental Health Block Grant provided $437 million to states in Fiscal 2003 (Directors report, 2003) and $436 million in 2005 (Lehmann, 2005). Most of this money continued to flow to community-based mental health services. Between 1990 and 1997, funds for state mental hospitals were substantially reduced whereas funds for community mental health programs increased by a proportion that was 26% above that of inflation. Unfortunately, state funding for mental health programs declined during this period from 2.1% to 1.8% of total state government expenditures—a 15% reduction (Lutterman & Hogan, 2000). This reduction has a major impact as in 2001, two-thirds of the funds for community mental health programs were being provided by state funds (Administration on Aging, 2001).

As a result of funding problems, cutbacks in programming have been made at many mental health centers. In 2002, the National Mental Health Association, an advocacy organization, argued that federal funding was becoming increasingly inadequate. In fact, while expenditures for health care continue to increase dramatically, the proportion of health care expenditures accounted for by mental health programs decreased between 1987 and 1997 (National Association of Mental Health Centers, 2004).

Mental health programs suffered further from the economic downturn that began in 2000. As tax revenues declined dramatically, states looked for ways to balance their budgets. Many states cut funding to mental health services. In Florida, one hospital district terminated its payments for psychotropic drugs for poor mental patients. Missouri closed down a psychiatric rehabilitation center. Other states such as Michigan began to close long-standing mental health facilities (Sherer, 2004). State cuts in Medicaid funding also had a negative impact on mental health programs as Medicaid funds are a large source of support for state mental health programs. The net result of these problems in funding can be seen in states such as California:

> In sum, California's community mental health system is a patchwork of state initiatives that ebb and flow with the will of the state's legislative and executive branches. County assumption of funding services beyond state realignment allocations appear to be unrealistic at best. Limited state and county allocations for home- and community-based services result in a relatively small number of service slots at the local level. Persons with psychiatric disabilities and their advocates (including family members) may not be aware of programs and services that should be available in the community. They also may not know what funds come into the county and where that money is spent, nor how local entities decide how to allocate some of their most precious resources (for example, crisis residential services, supported housing, or integrated services). [Stortz, 2003]

REFERENCES

Access to disability data. (2004). *Chartbook on mental health and disability.* Retrieved August 4, 2004, from http://www.infouse.com/disabilitydata/mentalhealth/4_phb

Administration on Aging. (2001). *Older Americans and mental health: Issues and opportunities.* Retrieved August 2, 2004, from http://www.protectassets.com/ssa/olderadultsandMH2001.pdf

Adult Health and Development Program. (2004). Retrieved July 18, 2004, from http://www.ahdp.org

American Association for Geriatric Psychiatry. (2004). *Health care professionals: Geriatric and mental health—the facts.* Retrieved August 2, 2004, from http://www.aagponline.org/prof/facts_mh.asp

Bratter, B. (1986). Peer counseling for older adults. *Generations, 10,* 49–50.

Bratter, B., & Freeman, E. (1990). The maturing of peer counseling. *Generations, 14,* 49–52.

Burns, B., Wagner, R., Taube, J., Magaziner, J., Permutt, T., & Landerman, R. (1993). Mental health service use by the elderly in nursing homes. *American Journal of Public Health, 83,* 331–337.

Butterfield, F. (2000). Prisons: The nation's new mental institutions. *Outreach Magazine.* Retrieved August 3, 2004, from http://www.psych-health.com/mental8.htm

Directors report. (2003, June). Retrieved August 3, 2004, from http://www.samhsa.gov.publications/allpubs/NMH-03-0154/default.asp

Family Service Agency of San Francisco. (2004). *The Senior Peer Counseling Program.* Retrieved August 3, 2004, from http://www.fsasf.org/services/SPC.htm

Fandetti, D., & Gelfand, D. (1978). Attitudes towards symptoms and services in the ethnic family and neighborhood. *American Journal of Orthopsychiatry, 48,* 477–486.

Glasscote, R., Biegel, A., Butterfield, A., Jr., Clark, E., Cox, B., Wiper, J. R., et al. (1976). *Old folks at homes.* Washington, DC: American Psychiatric Association and the Mental Health Association.

Grob, G. (2000). Mental health policy in 20th century America. In R. Manderscheid & M. Henderson (Eds.), *Mental health, United States, 2000.* Retrieved August 3, 2004, from http://www.mentalhealth.samhsa.gov/publications/allpubs.SMHA-3537/default.asp

Gulf Coast Jewish Family Services, Inc. (2004). *Mental health services.* Retrieved August 4, 2004, from http://www.gcjfs.org/svc-mental.htm

Katz, I. (2003). *Mental health in nursing homes: Lessons from late life depression.* Retrieved August 4, 2004, from http://www.mhaging/org/info/10-16-03-Katz.mh

Kornblatt, S., Cheng, S., & Chan, S. (2002). Best practices: The On Lok model of geriatric interdisciplinary care. *Journal of Gerontological Social Work, 40,* 15–22.

Lehmann, C. (2005). *APA pleased with budget boost for public mental health services*. Retrieved November 28, 2005, from http://pn.psychiatryonline.org/cgi/content/full/40/1/22-1

Levy, C. (2004, August 5). Home for mentally ill settles suit on coerced prostate surgery for $7.4 million. *New York Times,* p. A22.

Lutterman, T., & Hogan, M. (2000). State mental health agency controlled expenditures and revenues for mental health services. In R. Manderscheid & M. Henderson (Eds.), *Mental health, United States, 2000.* Retrieved August 3, 2004, from http://www.mentalhealth.samhsa.gov/publications/allpubs.SMHA-3537/default.asp

Michigan program links aging services with community mental health providers. (1990, December 7). *Older American Reports,* p. 474.

National Association of Mental Health Centers. (2004). *Community-based mental health services are under-funded.* Retrieved August 2, 2004, from http://www.namha.org/federal/appropriations/factsheet3.cfm

National Institute of Dental and Craniofacial Research. (2000). *Oral health in America: A report of the Surgeon General—Executive summary.* Rockville, MD: U.S. Department of Health and Human Services, National Institute of Dental and Craniofacial Research.

PACE (2004): Who we serve? Retrieved July 28, 2004, from http://www.nat-paceasson.org/content/research/who_served.asp

Rabins, P., Black, B., German, P., Tlassek-Wolfson, M., Penrod, J., Rabins, P., et al. (2000). The psychogeriatric assesssment and treatment in City Housing (PATCH) for elderly with mental illness in public housing: Getting through the crack in the door. *Archives of Psychiatric Nursing, 14,* 163–172.

Raschko, R. (1985). Systems integration at the program level: Aging and mental health. *Generations, 25,* 460–463.

Roca, R., Storer, D., Robbins, B., Tlasek, M., & Rabins, P. (1990). Psychogeriatric assessment and treatment in urban public housing. *Hospital and Community Psychiatry, 41,* 916–920.

Sherer, R. (2004). *A prescription for disaster: Cutbacks on mental health programs curb access to care.* Retrieved August 2, 2004, from http://www.psychiatrictimes.com/p040401a.html

Smyer, M., Shea, D., & Streit, A. (1994). The provision and use of mental health services in nursing homes: Results from the national medical expenditure survey. *American Journal of Public Health, 84,* 284–287.

Stortz, M. (2003). *A tale of two cities: Institutional and community-based mental health services in California since realignment in 1991.* Retrieved August 3, 2004, from http://www.pai-ca.org/pubs.540301.htm

Syracuse University School of Social Work. (1971). *Concerns in planning health services for the elderly.* Syracuse, NY: Author.

Vargas, C., Kramarow, E., & Yellowitz, J. (2001). *The oral health of older Americans.* Atlanta, GA: Centers for Disease Control.

Washington State, Mental Health Division. (2003). *Mental health best practices resource guide.* Retrieved August 6, 2004, from http://www.dshs.wa.gov.mentalhealth

Wei, W., Sambamoorthi, U., & Olfson, M. (2005). Use of psychotherapy for depression in older adults. *American Journal of Psychiatry, 162,* 711–717.

CHAPTER SEVEN

Transportation

Transportation programs can be designed to enable older persons to reach doctor's offices and hospitals. They also can be more wide-scale in their approach. As current OAA regulations define transportation services, they include:

> transporting older persons to and from community facilities and re-sources for purposes of acquiring/receiving services, to participate in activities or attend events in order to reduce isolation and promote successful independent living. Service may be provided through projects specially designed for older persons or through the utilization of public transportation systems or other modes of transportation. [U.S. Administration on Aging, 2004]

Transportation services are a vital element in community-based aging services, including day care centers, senior centers, mental health centers, and nutritional and educational programs. Developing transportation programs that ensure that older persons can access programs and services is feasible in many communities. Developing such programs that are available at all times for older persons who want to reduce their isolation by meeting friends or going to a movie or concert is a much more difficult process.

Most older Americans live in communities where there is inadequate public transit: 75% live in suburbs and in these suburban areas only 43% have any scheduled public transit within one-half mile of their homes (U.S. Senate Special Committee on Aging, 2003). As a result, older persons whose skills are seriously impaired continue to drive their own cars. The result is often tragic. Transportation-related fatalities rise significantly with age. Between 1991 and 1996, traffic fatalities were reduced overall, but not among older populations. Examined from a longer time perspective, between 1985 and 1996, fatalities increased 41% among drivers between the ages of 65 and 74 and 97% among drivers over the age of 75 (Hakamies-Blomquist, 2004). As the number of older Americans continues to increase, their representation in the driving population will also increase. In 2003, people over the age of 65 accounted for 14% of all drivers. By 2030, older people will comprise 25% of all drivers (U.S. Senate Special Committee on Aging, 2003). Despite their increased representation among drivers, 21% of individuals over the age of 65 do not drive. The reasons they do not drive include health problems, concerns about their safety, lack of a car, or personal preference to use other forms of transportation. The net result of this inability or unwillingness to drive is that 50% of older people stay home some days because they lack any transportation. This problem is most severe among minority elderly, suburban residents, and older persons living in rural areas (Surface Transportation Policy Project, 2004).

Various approaches to the transportation needs of urban, suburban, and rural elderly are thus required. To place the present thrust of transportation programs in an appropriate framework, we need to examine the goals of these services and the factors that impinge on realization of these goals.

OPTIONS

Transportation systems can vary in their extensiveness, their frequency of operation, and their ability to meet the individualized interests of potential consumers. In the language of transportation planning, these systems can be "demand-responsive," "need-responsive," or "desire-responsive." Whereas demand-responsive systems respond to individuals' calls for service, need-responsive systems attempt to service transportation requirements felt to be important to their maintenance of a satisfying life. The demands placed on transportation services by elderly individuals may be less than what they "need" for an independent, healthy lifestyle. Need-responsive systems are close to desire-responsive systems, and planners usually confine their analyses to these two groups.

The optimal transportation system for the elderly and the handicapped would be need-responsive, increasing the options of these populations for interactions with a range of individuals and programs. In densely populated areas, an inexpensive, properly designed mass transit system may enable the older person to reach a variety of important destinations. In suburban and rural areas with low density and dispersed services, a system responsive to the older person's needs is more difficult to implement.

MODELS

Aggregate trips taken by individuals to different sites, and the costs or subsidization that must be borne for each trip taken, are major factors in choosing transportation models appropriate to a community. As transit authorities around the country have discovered, public transit systems cannot be expected to run at a profit if fares are to be kept at a reasonable level. The growing understanding that public transit of any form needs to be subsidized has retarded its development in many areas. Unfortunately, many transit authorities attempting to stop the rise of deficits have become involved in a cycle of raising fares, resulting in a lower number of riders and subsequent fare increases. With each fare increase, the differential between the costs of mass transit and driving decreases, and increasing numbers of individuals therefore turn to their automobiles for commuting and pleasure trips. Transportation systems of all kinds must face the issue of the maximum subsidies that the community will tolerate and optimal methods for financing these subsidies.

FORMS OF TRANSPORTATION FOR THE ELDERLY

Mass Transit

During the 1960s and 1970s, an effort was made to encourage the use of existing mass transit facilities by the elderly. Under the 1974 National Mass Transit Assistance Act, the Urban Mass Transit Administration was authorized to allot funds for capital and operating costs of mass transit systems. Communities attempting to qualify for these funds were required to institute programs for the elderly that reduced fares in non-peak hours to no more than one-half of peak-hour fares. A number of major cities had already instituted this approach before the federal legislation was enacted. By 1974, 145 cities had already instituted half-fare programs (U.S. Department of Transportation, 1975).

The positive effects of programs for elderly riders have been demonstrated. These include increased use of the mass transit systems by the elderly to attend social activities and programs and to obtain medical care. Unfortunately, available studies do not reveal the reasons many elderly still refrain from using the transit system. The stress of the elderly concerning convenience and accessibility, rather than costs of transportation, may account for reduced ridership among older people, who may have to walk long distances to reach transit stops or take buses even to reach the subway. Having accomplished this task, they then must surmount obstacles posed by steps on buses or stairways in subway stations.

The Urban Mass Transportation Act (UMTA) specified that elderly and handicapped persons have the same rights to utilize mass transportation facilities and services as do other individuals. In 1975, regulations were issued requiring recipients of UMTA funds to build their facilities in a manner that would not create physical barriers for the elderly and handicapped. Installation of elevators at all new subway stations has been one major outgrowth of this requirement.

The physical barriers on buses are more difficult to overcome. In East Orange, New Jersey (Rinaldi, 1973), an escort service was provided during the early 1970s to help elderly individuals negotiate the steps of buses and other public transit barriers. In 1973, a negative report on this effort was issued. Despite the assistance made available by the escorts, the costs of this service were prohibitive. Costs were doubled, as fares were required for both the elderly person and the escort. The service was also not found to promote new trips by elderly individuals.

Regulations issued by the Department of Transportation required all new buses purchased with UMTA funds after September 1979 to have boarding ramps or hydraulic lifts, floor heights no more than 22 inches off the ground, and an ability to "kneel" to 18 inches. The regulations were rescinded in 1981, and local communities were allowed to demonstrate that they had made reasonable efforts to meet the needs of the elderly and the handicapped. Under the Americans with Disabilities Act passed in 1990, all new buses ordered must be accessible to people with disabilities. In major cities such as San Francisco, all buses now can kneel to allow elderly and disabled individuals easy boarding.

New Transportation Systems

Building public transportation systems is an extremely costly process, and these systems do not always provide the most direct route to a destination. In some cases, a bus trip to a medical center may require 50 minutes and a transfer of buses and cost $1.00. A taxicab ride to the same destination might take 10 minutes, cost $2.00, and travel door-to-door.

The problems involved in creating new transportation systems for the elderly are more complex than reductions in fares on existing mass transit facilities. Critical examination of the potential of new systems is necessary because of the increasingly decentralized living patterns of Americans. The Federal Aid to Highways Act of 1973 emphasized the need to take the mobility needs of rural elderly and handicapped into account in highway planning and improvements (U.S. Department of Transportation, 1976).

Through a major grant program (Section 5310), the Federal Transit Administration now provides funding to states "for the purpose of assisting private nonprofit groups in meeting the transportation needs of the elderly and persons with disabilities when the transportation service provided is unavailable, insufficient, or inappropriate to meeting these needs" (Federal Transit Administration, 2004). In Fiscal 2003, $90 million was allocated under this program. The funds are divided among the states based on the size of their older and disabled populations. In FY 2004, 58% of the funds were used by nonprofit groups for vans and 38% for buses at least 30 feet long (Federal Transit Administration, 2005). Although the Section 5310 funds have been valuable in all states, one estimate is that $350 million a year is required to meet the current needs of transportation systems for older persons and disabled persons (U.S. Senate Special Committee on Aging, 2003). The Section 5310 funds are supplemented in many communities by Older Americans Act Title III funds and purchase of care arrangements among individual social service agencies.

Substantial amounts of Title III funds have been channeled into transportation programs, although the AoA discourages the use of these monies for the purchase of vehicles. AoA officials fear that many agencies will not be able to afford the expenses of maintaining and operating these vehicles after using Title III funds to purchase them. The difficulties of meeting operating expenses is a common theme among organizations running extensive transportation efforts and facing mounting repair costs for heavily used vehicles. The costs of repairs plus high gasoline prices continue to make transportation an expensive service.

Obtaining adequate insurance at reasonable rates was previously a major headache for agencies attempting to implement transportation services for the elderly. In 1980, this major block to the expansion of transportation programs began to be resolved by new insurance ratings agreed upon by the federal government and the insurance industry. Under this new grouping, insurance ratings for vehicles owned by a program, or owned by employees or volunteers who transport the elderly, were placed midway between those for school buses and city buses. The new rates also provided excess liability insurance for the agency and the owner of the vehicle when transportation was provided for clients of a program. The excess liability was set at a low premium (Vehicle insurance rates, 1980). These new rates were the result of work on the part of the federal government and community groups to convince the insurance industry that the elderly were not more prone to injury when transported than other groups. In Janesville, Wisconsin, a transportation program staffed primarily by volunteers over the age of 55 uses a combination of the driver's own insurance (usually $300,000) and a blanket policy purchased by the program (Green, Associates, 1984). Section 5310 funds cannot be used for maintenance or insurance.

Fixed-route, fixed schedule services are available in a number of cities. These routes are most effective where large numbers of eligible riders live in close proximity. In Arlington, Virginia, 970 seniors live in four apartment complexes. As a result of this density, the local AAA has been successful in funding a local provider to implement a "Senior Loop." Using 16 passenger vans, the loop makes a continuous circuit during the middle of the day to transport residents to grocery stores (U.S. Senate Special Committee on Aging, 2003). In Jacksonville, Florida, the AAA has used Title III funds to purchase trips for older persons from providers. The providers include taxis, volunteers, local transit systems, and nonprofit groups. The rides must be reserved at least 24 hours in advance. In 2002, despite all of their efforts, the Jacksonville AAA estimated that for every individual served through this program, one had to wait for service (U.S. Senate Special Committee on Aging, 2003).

Many older people need a more flexible system. In Austin, Texas, the Reserve-A-Ride system charges $1 a ride for transportation to doctors or dentists, lawyers, banks, pharmacies, hair appointments, a friend in the hospital, volunteer work sites, or social engagements. The older person must call at least 24 hours in advance of the request date and riders are scheduled on a first-come, first-served basis.

An extensive transportation system is operated in Santa Barbara, California. Begun in 1987 with four vans, the Santa Barbara effort provided over 7,000 rides in August 1996. During Fiscal year 1995 the program provided 70,000 rides to 1,500 people who were unable to use available mass transit. As in Austin, a fee is charged for each ride and rides are provided on a first-come, first-served basis. The program operates on a 7-day-a-week schedule and provides curb-to-curb service. Drivers are not allowed to enter private homes or go past the lobby in nursing homes (U.S. Department of Transportation, 1997).

In Tennessee, the Mid-Cumberland Human Resources agency has implemented a "demand-responsive" system that offers rides to older people after 24 hours' notice. These rides are free to individuals over the age of 60 and 10,000 trips per month are now being undertaken through this program (Takas, 1996).

RIDERSHIP PROBLEMS

Encouraging frequent utilization of these transportation services is important in reducing the average cost per ride. Faced with the problems of financing expensive vans and then obtaining sufficient numbers of riders to keep subsidization at a reasonable level, it would appear that taxicab usage would be more economical and more convenient. Taxicab-based systems might also reduce any negative feelings that elderly residents have about riding special buses and would make use of existing dispatching systems.

In the early 1970s, a shared taxicab service was implemented in Arlington, Virginia. By 1975, this system had been abandoned on the basis of excessive costs (Kast, 1975). Arlington currently utilizes the STAR Assisted Transportation system. Selected taxicab drivers are trained to serve as escorts for older persons. They help these individuals from their house to the taxi and then to the door at their destination. Because of its cost, this Assisted Transportation System is only available for seniors going to doctors or other health care settings (U.S. Senate Special Committee on Aging, 2003). Aside from cost problems, many cab drivers may not want to pick up elderly passengers who live in poor inner-city or rural areas. The flexibility and convenience of the taxicab has thus been difficult to match with a program that is economical and efficient. "User side" subsidies do, however, appear to have strong support among older persons. Through its "Call 'N Ride" program, Montgomery County, Maryland, provides instituted taxi vouchers that low-income individuals over the age of 67 can purchase. Depending on the length of the ride, these vouchers can substantially reduce the cost (Montgomery County Maryland, 2004).

COORDINATION OF PROGRAMS

Many of the transportation programs for special groups are mandated under federal legislation. Medicaid legislation specifies that each state plan must include provisions for assuring the transportation of Medicaid recipients to and from medical services. This provision can be satisfied by reimbursement of recipients for their transportation costs. Title III of the OAA requires the provision of transportation for clients to and from nutrition sites if transportation is otherwise unavailable.

An indication of the proliferation of transportation programs was provided by a study that found 62 federal programs funding transportation efforts (U.S. General Accounting Office, 2003). Of these 62 programs, 23 were in the Department of Health and Human services, 15 in the Department of Labor, 8 in the Department of Education, and 6 in the Department of Transportation. The remaining 10 were scattered in a number of other agencies. In 2005, United We Ride found 37 federal programs that reimbursed consumers in different categories for their transportation expenses and 26 programs that funded the purchase and operation of vehicles or the contracting of transportation services with established providers. Coordination of individual agencies' efforts in order to pool resources for capital outlays and operating costs is one step that promises to reduce the constantly increasing financial burdens of these programs. In California, the local Transportation District provides 64% of the expenses for transportation programs in Marin County. The Transportation District also coordinates transportation programs for senior citizens, a medical transportation program, and a system of transportation for service and charitable organizations. The state of Georgia has appointed a Regional Transportation Coordinator for each of the state's 13 regions (U.S. Senate Special Committee on Aging, 2003).

At a more local level, Cleveland acted in the 1990s to create a more efficient transportation system for older people by consolidating four providers into one system that offers both fixed route and demand services (Three Ohio AAA's, 1990). In Detroit, the Commission on Jewish Eldercare Service has developed a coordinated system of transportation for seven different Jewish service agencies (U.S. Senate Special Committee on Aging, 2003).

FUTURE TRENDS

The transportation needs of older persons will continue to increase as the proportion of older persons living in suburban communities also increases. The emphasis on outpatient treatment for many health problems means that older persons will need to be able to reach their health providers on a regular basis. Many communities will attempt to provide fixed route transportation systems, but a more common model will be the type of system now in place in Arlington, Virginia.

The federal government is attempting to assist transportation programs through both subsidization of vouchers and capital assistance funds that allow organizations to buy vehicles. The Federal Transit Administration is placing a special emphasis on support for the development of special transit programs in rural areas. In these communities, 36% of the riders are elderly.

Even with this support, the provision of adequate transportation will remain a major issue for providers of services for older persons. The expenses associated with this service will not decrease, although the spiral in insurance premiums noted in the late 1970s has largely abated. Transportation will continue to consume a major portion of the budget of service agencies, even with proper coordination, and program planners must be aware of the costs and difficulties of providing adequate transportation.

For the elderly, we can expect transportation programs to remain demand-responsive rather than need-responsive. Although flexible schedules and route services may be officially available, priorities of shopping and medical trips may consume most of the van and bus capacity available in many areas. It is thus doubtful that any new public transportation system will be able to open up major new opportunities for elderly individuals to expand their range of activities. The realistic goals of transportation services should be to enable (1) formerly isolated elderly to reach the variety of agencies and programs now available, (2) elderly individuals to obtain the medical and mental health care they require, and (3) the elderly to undertake the necessary shopping trips to avoid doing without important goods. Visiting or attendance at cultural events requires a flexible and individualized service not within the resources of transportation systems presently in operation. Rural elderly and the increasing numbers of frail individuals over the age of 85 are two groups to whom specialized transportation services will need to be directed.

The goals mentioned are major, and their fulfillment will not be a simple task. Their attainment promises an improvement in the isolating conditions under which many elderly and handicapped now live, but it will remain an expensive effort. Subsidization of transportation services will always be necessary. Providing adequate transportation services may prove to be a major test of the general public's commitment to maintaining the network of services needed by older individuals.

REFERENCES

Federal Transit Administration. (2004). Transportation for elderly persons and persons with disabilities. Retrieved August 11, 2004, from http://www.fta.dot/grant_programs/specific_grant_programs/elderly_disabilities

Federal Transit Administration. (2005). *FY 2004 purchases by type of motor vehicle and program*. Retrieved November 28, 2005, from http://www.fta.dot.gov/files/t-10-11.xls

Green, Associates. (1984). *Use of volunteers in the transportation of elderly and handicapped persons*. Washington, DC: Urban Mass Transit Administration.

Hakamies-Blomquist, L. (2004). Safety of older persons in traffic. In *Transportation Research Board: Conference proceedings 27: Transportation in an aging society*. Retrieved August 12, 2004, from http://gulliver.trb.org/publications/conf/reports/cp_27.pdf

Kast, S. (1975, January 2). Arlington elderly about to lose those free rides. *Washington Star-News*, p. B-2.

Montgomery County, Maryland. (2004). *Call 'n Ride*. Retrieved August 24, 2004, from http://www.montogerycountymd.gov/APPS/DPTW/callnrideNEW/default.asp

Rinaldi, A. (1973). *Aid to senior citizens' mobility in East Orange, New Jersey: An escort service*. Millburn, NJ: National Council of Jewish Women.

Surface Transportation Policy Project. (2004). *Aging Americans: Stranded without options.* Retrieved July 28, 2004, from http://www.transact.org/library/reports_html/seniors/exec_sum.asp

Takas, T. (1996). *My father must stop driving.* Elder Law Fax, January 8.

Three Ohio AAA's use state funds for local initiatives. (1990). *Older American Reports, 14,* 399.

U.S. Administration on Aging. (2004). Retrieved from http://www.wiaaa.org/oaa_services/transportation_oaaservices.pdf

U.S. Department of Transportation. (1975). *Transportation for the elderly: The state of the art.* Washington, DC: U.S. Government Printing Office.

U.S. Department of Transportation. (1976). *Rural passenger transportation: Technology sharing.* Cambridge, MA: Transportation Systems Center.

U.S. Department of Transportation. (1997). *Transportation for a maturing society.* Washington, DC: Author.

U.S. General Accounting Office. (2003). *Transportation for disadvantaged populations.* Retrieved August 24, 2004, from http://www.gao.gov.new/items/d03697.pdf

U.S. Senate Special Committee on Aging. (2003). *Keeping America's seniors moving: Examining ways to improve senior transportation, July 21.* Washington, DC: U.S. Government Printing Office.

Vehicle insurance rates lowered for elderly programs. (1980). *Older American Reports, 4,* 4.

CHAPTER EIGHT

Crime and Legal Assistance Programs

Whereas programs related to crime attempt to protect the older adult from victimization, many of the legal services stressed in aging attempt to protect the elderly from harming themselves. Legal services have increased since they became the focus of attention at the 1971 White House Conference on Aging and in the 1975 amendments to the OAA.

Legal programs for older persons are diverse in nature. Even the laws on guardianship and protective services differ from state to state. Because it is impossible to cover all of these rapidly growing and changing programs, this chapter will provide an overview of the types of programs now in existence.

THE ELDERLY AND CRIME

Concerns and Figures

Concern about crimes against the elderly has intensified in recent years. Reports of elderly people being mugged and murdered frequently make front-page headlines. In 1977, the report of a Brooklyn, New York, couple who committed suicide after leaving a note stating that death was better than living in continual fear received major coverage throughout the United States. It remains unclear, however, whether the reality of the crime rate matches the concern that it raises among older people or in the media.

Data collected on crimes committed against elderly victims are imprecise, as are criminal statistics in general. The FBI compiles its widely relied-upon statistics from incidents of crime reported to local police departments, which have varied reporting requirements. There is also a widespread belief that older individuals fear either dealing with the police or retaliation by attackers who live in the neighborhood, and therefore often avoid reporting crimes against them. Finally, if a crime is reported to the police, the age of the victim is not always recorded.

Patterns of Crime

The rates of criminal acts perpetrated against the elderly are different from those perpetrated against younger individuals. Property crimes, not violence, accounts for the largest proportion of crimes against older persons. Although thefts comprise only 3% of the crimes against individuals age 12–49, they comprise 20% of the crimes committed against older persons (U.S. Department of Justice, Bureau of Justice Statistics, 2005a). In 2004, robberies of persons over the age of 65 occurred at a rate of .3/1,000 compared to the highest rate of 4.8/1,000 among individuals aged 16–19 (Catalano, 2005). Because many older persons find it difficult to drive or access public transportation, they restrict their activities. Many of the attacks against older individuals occur close to their homes because they have problems obtaining adequate transportation to other communities.

The consequences of crime can be more severe for people over the age of 65 than they are for younger individuals. Physical injuries may prove incapacitating for a long period. The psychological trauma resulting from being a victim of crime may result in the older person withdrawing from many social activities (Asheville, N.C. Police Department, 2004). As Table 8.1 indicates, individuals are less likely to be victims of most categories of crime after the age of 19, with the lowest rates in all categories among individuals over age 65. It can be argued that the number of crimes against older persons would be more extensive if many elderly did not remain at home in the evening, thus also restricting their involvement in the social life of the community.

Vulnerability

A low income makes it difficult for many older persons to recoup from robbery, and it also makes them susceptible to confidence games that hold out the promise of quick wealth. Older individuals faced with the threat of violence may not have the physical strength to fight off a potential attacker, and thus may be viewed as easy victims. The elderly also tend to reside in areas of the city where unemployment and general social problems abound. Many of these elderly residents receive their checks for Social Security, SSI, or pensions on fixed dates of each month. These dates

TABLE 8.1 Victim Rates for Persons 12 and Over by Type of Crime and Age of Victims, 2002

| | Crimes of Violence/1,000 | | | | | | |
| | Age | | | | | | |
	12–15	16–19	20–24	25–34	35–49	50–64	65+
All personal crimes	45.3	58.8	49.0	26.8	18.8	11.0	4.0
Violence	44.4	58.2	47.4	26.3	18.1	11.0	3.4
Robbery	3.0	4.0	4.7	2.8	1.5	1.6	1.0
Assault	39.3	48.6	39.8	22.8	16.1	8.9	2.2
Simple	34.3	36.7	29.7	12.9	9.4	5.7	1.3

Source: U.S. Department of Justice, Bureau of Justice Statistics, 2002.

are often common knowledge in the neighborhood and become red-letter days for attackers. The development of a system of direct deposit of checks is helping to reduce this problem. The elderly are also easy prey for attackers because they often live alone and go out shopping by themselves rather than in groups.

Confidence Schemes

In addition to the physical weakness and living habits that increase the vulnerability of the elderly to violent crime, the American aged have a number of other characteristics that make them "marks" for consumer fraud. Especially important is their fear of growing older and of the loss in functioning they assume will be part of aging. Devices that promise to prevent or repair losses in hearing or vision may be especially attractive to older adults, and those who suffer from chronic illnesses frequently jump at the opportunity to purchase medications that promise to relieve their pain. All of these factors are most at play among the less-educated elderly. Older individuals with more education show less interest in over-priced merchandise and less susceptibility to fraudulent schemes.

A common of confidence game is the "pigeon drop." In this scheme, someone approaches an elderly person on the street and informs him or her that a bag of money has been found. The money will be shared if the older person shows good faith by going to the bank and withdrawing some funds, which will be held by an attorney until the bag of money is legally released to them.Once given the money, the con artist disappears. Other con games are variations on this theme, which promise the elderly some easy reward for providing some of their funds as a sign of good faith or as security.

Unscrupulous retailers and salespeople who encourage the elderly to buy items that are unnecessary, inadequate, or overpriced engage in a second form of fraud. The most common consumer frauds perpetuated against the aged involve hearing aids, eyeglasses, funeral arrangements, dentures, and health insurance. In many cases, the elderly are encouraged to buy prosthetics such as hearing aids, that will not make up for their auditory losses or are overpriced. Some major insurance companies have been sued for making false claims about life insurance policies they marketed to older persons.

Telemarketing has also made it easier to reach seniors and perpetrate these frauds. In addition to bogus products, telemarketing of fraudulent home repair and cleaning frauds is common. In these schemes, services are contracted for but not delivered adequately by the provider. The estimate is that 80% of the victims of telemarketing frauds have been over the age of 65 (U.S. Senate Special Committee on Aging, 2000).

Living alone, and often isolated, older men and women can fall prey to individuals who befriend them:

> I met Marvin Norby several years ago when he purchased a car that my grandson had for sale that was parked in my driveway. Marvin came to my house to pay for the car and asked if he could visit me. And he seemed nice, so I said that would be fine. In a few days, Marvin brought some muffins over and we visited, and then he started coming over more frequently.
>
> Marvin told me that he had inherited a house in Tacoma and he was preparing the house for sale, but he needed funds to fix it up. I loaned him $2,000 to do some of the work. Marvin told me I would get my money back when the house sold. Marvin also told me that he had put my name on the deed to the house and I would be sure to get my money back.
>
> Marvin kept asking for more and more money and I kept giving him more. I gave him almost $106,000. In the meantime Marvin also needed money for different things like surgery that he had to have, so I helped him with all he asked for. [U.S. Senate, Special Committee on Aging, 2000]

Many frauds of this kind go unreported. Older persons often do not realize that these frauds are a crime and have no information about services that are available. Some states have developed programs to create more awareness about common frauds. Arizona has established Elder Fraud Prevention Teams that make presentations and conduct events to alert seniors and their families about potential frauds. Kentucky offers a Senior Crime College consisting of 2½-hour educational sessions on how to avoid victimization and who to call if you are victimized. In one 2-year period, the program attracted more than 10,000 attendees (U.S. Department of Justice, 2000).

An increasing problem is Internet fraud. With no controls on Web sites, it is difficult to assess the quality or reliability of specific sites. Sites that offer travel services, employment services, and get-rich quick schemes have become subjects of an increasing number of complaints to consumer affairs offices. In Oregon, problems with Internet sites had become the ninth most reported type of complaint by 1999 (U.S. Senate Special Committee on Aging, 2000). Older persons are particularly vulnerable to Internet sites that offer low-cost prescriptions. Even if these medications are delivered as promised, there is no guarantee as to their quality.

CRIME PREVENTION AND ASSISTANCE

Robberies, attacks, consumer frauds, and confidence swindles can beset the elderly. Because victimization can take so many forms, the programs that have been devised to protect the victims are also extensive. They are run under a variety of auspices, including general or special units of the Police Department. Some programs are operated by the local Area Agency on Aging or a social service agency.

Educational Programs

Educational programs about crime for older persons focus on the avoidance of street crimes and confidence swindles. A second type of program related to crime prevention encourages increased cohesion in the community and the implementation of support services, such as an escort service, or a neighborhood watch effort. The police department in Atlanta, Georgia, has developed a specific neighborhood watch program oriented to older residents. Using a "buddy system," neighbors check up on each other and escort each other to the doctor's office or the market. The buddies also watch each other's homes when neighbors are away (National Crime Prevention Council, 2004). Finally, most areas now have some form of victim assistance program that provides both financial compensation and counseling to victims of crime.

At the national level, AARP, the International Association of Chiefs of Police, and the National Sheriff's Association have combined to develop the Triad program. Triad forms local advisory councils consisting of law enforcement agents, providers, and older individuals to discuss and recommend programs that will reduce crimes against older persons. With the help of volunteers, Triad can carry out a variety of activities. Triad members can conduct surveys of crime-related concerns among older people and prepare lists of available legal services. In addition, they can plan new crime prevention programs for older persons, foster better communication between the community and law enforcement agencies, and recruit seniors as volunteers in crime prevention efforts (*The tried solution,* 2004). In Philadelphia, North West Victims Services (NWVS) conducts programs at senior centers on how to prevent fraud. NWVS also visits local banks as part of its Bank Session Project. During these visits, seniors are counseled about safe banking habits and general safety. Between 1990 and 1991, 2,000 older people were counseled at 10 banks (Tomz & McGill, 1997). In Baltimore, Maryland, the mayor's office has developed videotapes dealing with assault, robbery, and burglaries. These tapes concentrate on techniques that can be used when the individual is confronted with these crimes.

In Los Angeles, the Interagency Task Force on Crime against the Elderly was formed from the law enforcement agencies, the Area Agencies on Aging, social service agencies, libraries, and educational institutions in the area to design educational programs dealing with victimization of the elderly. The task force's efforts have included the use of television and radio announcements. California has also attempted, through its Consumer Information and Protection Program for Seniors, to provide education for the elderly on prevalent types of consumer fraud. Oklahoma has established an Office of Legal Rights. This office offers a variety of services including talks around the state on legal issues that concern older individuals as well as consultations to attorneys, paralegals, and advocacy groups about these issues (Legal Services Developer, n.d.).

Security Programs

In many areas with a high concentration of elderly, educational efforts have been combined with increased security measures. The Law Enforcement Assistance Administration (LEAA) funded a project in Syracuse, New York, to establish security units in eight low-income elderly housing projects. In Plainfield, New Jersey, a $6,000 program was developed to control access into senior housing units through the use of closed-circuit TV systems. In South Bend, Indiana, $3,000 was spent for the installation of door locks for elderly residents who could not afford them. The South Bend police operated this project.

The federally funded "Blow the Whistle on Crime" program made efforts to provide whistles to individuals in over 300 cities. In the Crown Heights section of Brooklyn and in high-crime areas of Milwaukee, Wisconsin, and Wilmington, Delaware, "security aides" provided escort services for the elderly. The Wilmington program utilized both older individuals and teenagers as escorts. With funding cuts in fiscal 1982 and the disappearance of LEAA as an independent agency, the emphasis became focused on technical assistance through dissemination of materials rather than direct program funding.

Victim Assistance

A final group of programs is aimed at providing assistance to individuals who have been the victims of crime. Many of these programs began with funding through the 1984 Victims of Crime Act. A variety of services are provided through these programs, ranging from emergency assistance to counseling and help with the legal system or obtaining compensation due crime victims. A survey of 319 victim assistance programs indicated that the most common form of assistance was information about the legal rights of victims. Among individuals served, 8% were over the age of 65 (McEwen, 1995). In Santa Ana, California, the victim assistance program has a Senior Victim of Crime Specialist who may go to an older person's home to offer help. In Minneapolis-St. Paul, the program staff visits the homes of older victims of crime and boards up damaged windows and secures damaged doors (Tomz & McGill, 1997). In the Hartford, Connecticut, area, a Senior Victim Assistance Program provides a variety of services for older persons who have been victims of crime, including counseling and advocacy, home visits, and information about financial compensation for violent crimes (Senior Victim Assistance Program, 2004).

"Victim centers" in major cities serve all age groups and are often located within police departments. In Asheville, North Carolina, the police department offers a program of Older Adult Victim Services. Since 1997 the program has helped almost 1,600 older and disabled individuals. As in Connecticut, an advocate visits the person's home or the hospital, provides counseling and information about ongoing investigation of the crime, and supplies referral to service providers (Asheville, N.C. Police Department, 2004). Many elderly crime victims are reluctant to serve as witnesses. To cope with this problem, there are also "witness centers" in conjunction with the local courts. The witness is informed about court procedures and provided with necessary services, such as transportation. The centers will provide protection for witnesses if necessary.

The Victims of Crime Act, passed in 1984, has helped to fund state compensation and victim assistance programs throughout the country. The Act is administered through the Office for Victims of Crime at the U.S. Department of Justice. This office provides funds to states for both victim compensation and victim assistance. The funds to compensate victims for their losses and injuries vary across the country but range from $10,000 to $25,000. These funds are allocated only if private insurance and restitution from the offenders is inadequate (U.S. Department of

Justice, Office for Victims of Crime, 2004). The victim assistance monies fund such efforts as counseling and referral. Over $3 billion had been allocated for these efforts between fiscal 1986 and 2003 (U.S. Department of Justice, Office for Victims of Crime, 2004). Unfortunately, many elderly people find that they are not reimbursed by insurance for what they lose as a result of victimization. Many states have not instituted victim compensation laws that provide reimbursement for the costs sustained by all individuals. The state-by-state variation in these victim compensation laws is great. The maximum amount of compensation for medical expenses or loss of earnings varies, as does the maximum time within which a victim may file a claim.

Despite all of this activity, the effectiveness of these programs is not yet clear. The loss of a feeling of community and the general fear that pervade many American cities is still strong. This fear can also be found among suburban elderly even if they have not personally experienced criminal victimization (Cantor, Brook, & Mellor, 1986). Crime rates dropped significantly in recent years. Between 1994 and 2002, violent crimes declined to their lowest level ever and property crime rates continued a 20-year decline (U.S. Department of Justice, Bureau of Justice Statistics, 2005b). It remains unclear whether this reduction is the result of new punitive policies that stress longer prison sentences or fewer numbers of younger individuals, the group most likely to commit crimes. It is also unclear whether older persons feel any more secure as a result of these changes in reported crimes.

LEGAL REPRESENTATION

As services for this population have increased, the elderly have become more involved with a variety of public and private bureaucracies that determine their eligibility for these programs. Disputes about eligibility may necessitate legal representation. For older people, legal issues that most often arise are questions about Social Security and SSI benefits, landlord–tenant disputes, Medicare claims, food stamp certification, and wills and probates.

There is little doubt that the elderly have not received adequate legal assistance, partially because lawyers are not likely to earn high fees working with them. Many older persons also remain unaware of their legal rights, or are afraid of dealing with lawyers, just as they do not report crimes out of fear of dealing with the police. Even elderly individuals who do have higher educational backgrounds and who are more confident about legal transactions may lack the transportation necessary to reach a lawyer's office.

Legal representation for the elderly has begun to improve in recent years, mainly through the efforts of the Legal Services Corporation (LSC), authorized under federal legislation in 1975. This corporation is an independent successor to the poverty law program that existed within the now-defunct Office of Economic Opportunity. The LSC has lawyers in offices throughout the country and services all individuals, including the elderly who fall below the federal poverty level. In 2002, the LSC was operating 179 local programs throughout the United States (Legal Services Corporation, 2004). Specialized programs for the elderly have been supported by funds from a variety of federal programs, and foundations have increased legal representation for the elderly. The LSC and the AoA have provided support to the National Senior Citizens Law Center (NSCLC). The NSCLC has three major priorities: (1) advocacy for the elderly poor, (2) litigation on issues of access and procedures, and (3) training, informing, and assisting local advocates for the elderly (National Senior Citizens Law Center, 2004).

Approximately 11% of Legal Services Corporation clients are over the age of 60. The cases these older clients bring to court usually involve questions of eligibility for government benefits. The threat of legal action is also helpful in situations where private pension plans contain major loopholes and possibilities of abuse by employers. In one case, a truck driver for a major supermarket chain retired after 34 years of work, expecting a pension of $300 a month. When his first check arrived, he found that it was for only $250. The employer informed him that his pension had been reduced because he retired a month too early, even though his retirement date was advised by an official of the firm. A student at George Washington University Law School wrote to the supermarket chain about the problem. After 2 months, the retired driver received a check for $1,200, an apology from the company for the mistaken advice, and credit for the additional month.

Funding for the LSC has been cut substantially, reducing the availability of personnel and the type of cases the agency could handle. LSC is now ineligible to bring class action suits and must involve itself only with individual cases. The budget reductions resulted in 300,000 fewer cases being handled by LSC in 1996 and the closing of 300 offices. In 2004, LSC funded 143 programs across the country staffed by 3,700 attorneys (Barnett, 2004).

Though the efforts of the LSC and the NSCLC are admirable, these organizations alone are unable to provide sufficient legal representation to serve the multiple needs of the elderly. Some law schools have set up special clinics to serve the elderly, and the numbers of lawyers working in the area of estate planning and benefits is increasing. One innovative approach to meeting the legal representation needs of older persons is the

Legal Hotline. The first such hotlines were developed in 1985 by the Legal Counsel for the Elderly. Attorneys are paid a per diem rate to offer legal information or advice to a caller. They can also refer the caller to a publicly funded legal program or a program that offers services for a reduced fee. If the attorney decides that the caller's problem is not a legal problem, he or she may refer the older person to a local social service agency (Kolasa & Soto, 1990). Legal hotlines may be funded through organizations such as AARP or through community organizations using AoA funding.

Many AAAs maintain lists of lawyers in their area. Some states, however, go beyond this basic service. The state of Maine operates a Legal Services for the Elderly program that offers legal services for low-income persons over the age of 60.

The hotlines overcome transportation problems facing the elderly and help older persons define problems more carefully without facing major legal fees (Kolasa & Soto, 1990). There have been some problems with the hotlines. Most prominent has been high turnover rates among the staffing attorneys. Hotlines have also had difficulty working with hearing-impaired older callers (Porter & Affeldt, 1990).

Pro bono representation is now a policy of the American Bar Association, but attempts to specify the amount of time lawyers should donate to clients have been resisted. Although efforts are being made to increase lawyers' gratis representation of the elderly, it is likely that para-legal counselors will undertake much of the increased legal counseling.

Legal services were classified as one of the three priorities in the 1973 OAA amendments. As part of its plan for the aging, each state was required to show that the Area Agencies on Aging (AAAs) were contracting for legal services while making efforts to involve private bar organizations in legal services at reduced rates or free. The emphasis on legal services was deleted from the 1981 amendments in line with the concept that localities should exercise control of programs.

Some of the funds for legal services have been allotted to the ombudsman programs. In fiscal 2001, 596 ombudsman programs funded by a combination of federal and nonfederal funds were operational. The 1987 OAA amendments included a specific authorization of $20 million for the ombudsman program and specific guidelines for establishing a long-term care ombudsman program with the State Offices on Aging. The State Office on Aging, or contractor, is charged with using the ombudsman program to investigate complaints by residents of long-term care facilities and to establish procedures for access by the ombudsman to these facilities. The amendments also prohibit retaliation by a long-term care facility against an individual or employee who files a complaint or provides information to an ombudsman. In FY 2001, $60 million was being spent on ombudsman programs for seniors around the country. Of this total, 60% was from federal funds and the remainder from non-federal sources, primarily state funds (Administration on Aging, 2001). In addition to approximately 1,000 full-time equivalent employees, 13,000 certified and non-certified volunteers respond to complaints brought to their attention. An analysis of complaints about nursing home care revealed an increase in the number of complaints to ombudsmen from 145,000 in 1997 to 186,000 in 2000 (Office of the Inspector General, n.d.).

PROTECTIVE SERVICES

Whereas in many cases legal representation of an elderly person can increase the person's self-sufficiency, protective service measures remove many of the rights an individual has to make his or her own decisions. Elderly persons who are thought to be unable to manage their personal or financial affairs in their own best interests are subject to the imposition of protective services designed to protect them from themselves and from unscrupulous third parties (Horstman, 1977).

Elements of Protective Services

Protective services have two major components: (1) intensive services provided, with the individuals' consent, to those who appear to need major supportive assistance, and (2) services provided for individuals after a hearing, without their consent, which involve "legally enforced supervision of guardianship which, temporarily depriving the client of certain rights, enables an agency to assist the person" (Regan & Springer, 1977, p. 4). These services and guardianship may be imposed on individuals of any age, but the concept of protective services has been most widely applied to individuals over 60.

Recipients

We can define the type of person for whom protective services might be appropriate by examining an individual case.

> Mr. E., 73, a tall, powerfully built man with no surviving family, formerly a skilled iron worker, had become settled, but not rooted, in one area of town after an early adulthood of country-wide transiency. He had never married but was proud of earlier feminine conquests. Inarticulate, having had a large investment in his body image, he now lacked the kind of strengths that formerly had helped him achieve his goals. With a foreign upbringing and little formal

education, Mr. E. was now frustrated by the ravages of illness and old age. He reacted with extreme intolerance of others, suspicion, and severe verbal abusiveness. At the point of referral, Mr. E. was in grave danger of dying and was thwarting efforts of interested agencies to induce him to accept proper medical attention through hospitalization. Despite his cleanliness of person, his disabilities had affected the maintenance of his small apartment, which was cluttered and dirty. A friendship of 20 years with a male friend indicated some underlying capacity for human attachment. The grave medical problems were compounded by the limitations of an income of $105 monthly from Social Security (Wasser, 1974, pp. 103–114).

Mr. E. can obviously benefit from many forms of assistance, including a variety of personal services. He may also be one of the 25% of the elderly often estimated to have major mental health problems.

During the famous social experiment in protective services at the Benjamin Rose Institute of Cleveland, individuals such as Mr. E. were provided with intensive casework assistance from experienced social workers with master's degrees in social work. These social workers functioned under one overriding directive: "Do, or get others to do, whatever is necessary to meet the needs of the situation" (Blenkner, Bloom, Nielsen, & Weber, 1974, p. 68). In order to be effective, the social workers had to utilize a variety of concomitant services needed by clients of the protective services program. These included financial assistance, medical evaluations, home aides, and psychiatric consultation. In 20% of the cases, legal consultation was utilized; in 12%, guardianship proceedings were instituted and completed. The Benjamin Rose program provides a model for the types of assistance that protective services might supply, its basic assumption being that clients of the program require more intensive assistance than is normally provided by most agencies.

GUARDIANSHIP

Guardianship for older persons has become more common, but it is difficult to obtain reliable data on the exact numbers of guardianships now in place. The report that Michigan alone had 100,000 guardianships in 2000 indicates the possibility of an extensive number across the country (U.S. Senate Special Committee on Aging, 2003). Whatever the actual number of existing guardianships, the trends certainly point to higher numbers in upcoming years. Between 1992 and 1997, the number of guardianships granted in New York increased from 15,000 to 32,000 (U.S. Senate Special Committee on Aging, 2003). Contemporary legal guidelines for guardianship and commitment are inadequate. The complex questions raised by protective services have been outlined by Blenkner and colleagues (1974):

1. If the services provided to an individual such as Mr. E. are inadequate and are resisted by Mr. E., who should have the right to define Mr. E. as a problem and deprive him of his ability to make decisions?
2. If older persons resist services, does provision of services against their will provide them with assistance, or merely satisfy the "psychological discomfort" of the social worker?
3. Is providing protective services the answer to the problems of Mr. E., or is the real issue for the elderly the conditions that are imposed on them, and under which they are forced to live?
4. If the proposed solution to Mr. E.'s problems is placement in a long-term care setting, will this solve the problems for the family and neighbors upset by his behavior, but be destructive to his own personal functioning?
5. Can any services, whether voluntary or imposed, help many of the individuals who come under the wing of protective services improve to a "normal" functioning level?

Even if answers to these questions affirm the need for protective services, there remains the necessity of careful criteria for legal intervention models. There are increased signs of an understanding of the complexity and importance of guardianship. Among the eligible supportive services included in Title III of the 1992 OAA amendments are "representation in guardianship proceedings by older individuals who seek to become guardians . . . and information and training for individuals who are or may become guardians . . ." [Sec. 312].

Consequences of Guardianship

An individual placed under guardianship can suffer a variety of losses. These include the right to sue, charge purchases, engage in contracts, deed property, marry, divorce, open a bank account, or vote. In some states, the individual's eligibility for program benefits, including Medicare and pensions, will come under scrutiny when a guardian is appointed.

An incompetent is defined traditionally as one who by reason of mental illness, drunkenness, drug addiction, or old age is incapable of self-care, of managing business, or of exercising family responsibilities, or as one who is liable to dissipate an estate or become the victim of designing persons (Regan & Springer, 1977). In most states, the individual must be declared incompetent in order for a guardian to be appointed. Vague bases for declarations of incompetence such as "old age" have contributed to the abuses now associated with the protective services approach. Despite these changes, there are still variations across states in the procedures required in guardianship hearings. In 15 states, the presence of the older person being considered for guardianship is mandatory. Many other states dispense with the older person's attendance in the "best interest of the clients." On a national basis, only 8% of older people actually attend the guardianship proceedings in which they are involved. Guardianships can also be used in emergency situations.

Incapacity is defined as the inability of the person to care for his or her person or property or the imminent danger to the person of physical harm or material waste. This is the standard for making decisions about the need for guardianship. The criteria for determining incapacity range from "clear and convincing" evidence to vaguer standards that stress the "best interests of the ward." In over half of the 34 states, a medical examination is required, and 14 states include a psychological examination. Minnesota employs a more comprehensive approach, requiring separate evaluations by a physician, a psychologist, and a social worker with recommendations about the type of guardianship best suited for the individual.

In some states, this interdisciplinary approach has been formalized through the development of Geriatric Evaluation Services (GES). The GES evaluates clients being considered for commitment to a mental hospital, appointment of a conservator, emergency protective services, or protective placements. In many of the states, the terms "guardian" and "conservator" are used interchangeably, and only careful reading of the statutes indicates the responsibility of the individual appointed by the court. One-third of the states initially prefer to utilize an adult child, parent, or relative of the person as a guardian. If none of these choices is available, then a public guardian is called upon. In 20 states, a specific state or county agency is designated in the legislation as the public guardian of the older person. In seven states, the ward has an opportunity to participate in the selection of the guardian.

In the view of Schmidt, Miller, Bell, and New (1981), those states that appoint a public agency providing services to the ward as a guardian are developing a conflict of interest. The agency's priority may be efficient and low-cost service delivery rather than protection of an individual. Seventeen states have the same agency providing services and acting as a guardian. Few of the states explicitly mention the funding of the guardian, and 20 of the 34 states make some provision for review of the guardianship. These alterations, while not sufficient, are clear evidence of changes in philosophy concerning protective services and guardianship.

The guardianship-conservator model is long term in nature. There is, however, a rationale for an emergency intervention model for individuals whose needs are immediate or expected to be temporary. In most states, individuals believed to be dangerous to themselves and others may be confined for a period that averages 72 hours. After that time, a formal hearing must be held to determine whether an individual should be committed for a longer period. In Maryland, three criteria must be evident before individuals can be committed to a state mental facility: the individuals must (1) be dangerous to themselves or the community, (2) require inpatient treatment, and (3) be mentally ill.

Alternatives to long-term commitment have not existed until recently and have not always been explored by protective service workers. Alternative settings were a major point in the landmark *Lake v. Cameron* (1966) decision, in which the Washington D.C. Court of Appeals ruled that Mrs. Lake could not be held in St. Elizabeth's Hospital unless all other possible less restrictive alternatives were explored. Unfortunately for Mrs. Lake, no alternatives available at that time (1966) were deemed appropriate, and she was remanded to St. Elizabeth's.

Changes in Protective Services

As guardianship has become more utilized around the country, the potential for abuse of this system has become apparent. Abuse can be found on the part of family members who institute guardianship proceedings to obtain the financial resources of their elderly relatives, or lawyers who misuse funds after being appointed as guardians. A number of major changes are being promoted throughout the country to prevent undue restriction of the civil rights of the elderly. These include:

1. Changes in the law to redefine competency according to the level at which an individual is capable of functioning, rather than by a vague medical diagnosis;
2. requirements that the individual be informed of the importance of guardianship hearings, the right to counsel, and the right to cross-examine witnesses. It is interesting to note that one study in Los Angeles found that in only 2% of the guardianship hearings was counsel present for the subject. In Ohio, a negative correlation of .94 was found between representation by counsel and decisions to commit an individual to a long-term care institution (U.S. Senate Special Committee on Aging, 2003).
3. legislation to authorize a full range of protective social services throughout the country; and
4. establishment of a system of public guardianship for people without private guardian resources.

Horstman (1977) argued for a "bill of rights" for all aged people that would define their constitutional rights in relation to confinement. Under his plan, confinement would be utilized only when the following five conditions were present:

1. The individual had been declared mentally incompetent to determine the viability of seeking or refusing treatment, and
2. Less restrictive alternatives to total institutionalization have been fully explored and found to be inadequate to protect and maintain the individual, and
3. The individual is unable to live safely in freedom either by himself or with the assistance of willing and responsible family members or friends, and
4. The individual is untreatable, and
5. Institutionalization is in the individual's best interest (p. 288).

It could be argued that a nationwide development of protective services might cut down the need for guardianship or commitment hearings. The Benjamin Rose Institute study stressed caution in aggressively expanding protective services. The research did not show significant differences on a number of measures between individuals in the experimental and control groups. As summed up by Blenkner, Bloom, Wasser, and Nielsen (1971):

> For the participant, himself, however, there was no significant impact with respect to increased competence or slowed deterioration and greater contentment or lessened disturbance. Furthermore, although he was more "protected," the participant was no less likely to die when given protective services than when left to the usual and limited services of the community. In fact, the findings on functional competence together with those on death and institutionalization force consideration of the hypothesis that intensive service with a heavy reliance on institutional care may actually accelerate decline. [p. 494]

This negative evaluation placed a brake on the development of protective services and raised important questions in many social workers' minds about the degree to which the development of extensive services promoted dependency of the aged on the worker. A reanalysis by a new group of researchers at the Benjamin Rose Institute (Bigot, Demling, Shuman, & Schur, 1978) indicates, however, that the original staff may have underestimated the positive effects of the intensive social work services. The federally funded "channeling" demonstration provided a single point of access to coordinated services. Reports on the effects of this project were released in 1986. These data raise again the issue of whether extensive services to older persons may not produce dependency and reduce functioning levels (Mathematica Policy Research, 1986). The positive and negative effects of protective social casework services offered by agencies remains unclear. The effects of legal procedures for the elderly that remove their rights are much clearer in their negative implications. Legislative enactments as outlined by Regan and Springer (1977) will afford due process for the elderly and restrict the power to unduly remove their civil liberties. These legislative revisions should be a prime concern for advocates of aging programs and practitioners in aging.

Elder Abuse

In recent years abuse and neglect of older persons has become a major topic of concern for protective service workers. Elder abuse is defined by the Administration on Aging (1998) as including physical, psychological, and financial abuse and neglect.

The 1984 amendments to the OAA required AAAs to assess the need for elder abuse services in their jurisdictions, and the 1987 amendments authorized a $5 million program of grants for elder abuse services and education. Title VII of the 1992 OAA amendments authorized at least $15 million for elder abuse programs. These funds were earmarked for education about elder abuse, receipt of reports about elder abuse, outreach to older persons who may be the victims of elder abuse, and referrals of complaints about elder abuse to law enforcement agencies [Sec. 705(a)(6)].

Reported elder abuse cases numbered 117,000 in 1986 but had increased to 551,011 in 1996. Whatever the reported figures, it is estimated that four times as many cases of elder abuse are unreported as reported (Administration on Aging, 2004). Partly because of the stigmatized behavior it represents, the actual prevalence of elder abuse and neglect remains in question. The best estimate is between 800,000 and 1.8 million actual cases but even the higher figure may be too low (National Center on Elder Abuse, 1999). Self-neglect appears to be the most common problem (58.5%), followed by physical abuse (15.7%), and financial exploitation (12.3%). Among the reported cases of abuse, 65% of the abused older persons were White, 21.4% African American, and 9.6% Latino (Administration on Aging, 1998). In 1996, the number of cases of elder abuse reported among the population over the age of 80 were two to three times the proportion of this age group in the general population. Sadly, two-thirds of the abuse perpetrators were adult children or spouses (Administration on Aging, 2004). The lack of adequate numbers of research studies has severely hampered the effort to come to grips with the real dimensions of the elder abuse problem in the United States.

By 1997, 42 states had passed legislation requiring professionals to report elder abuse. In 1990, Mississippi enacted legislation making elder abuse and neglect in nursing homes and hospitals a felony offense (NAR-CEA Exchange, 1990). Pennsylvania has enacted a law providing legal protection for individuals who report suspected elder abuse. This diversity in response across states remains one of the major problems in combating elder abuse. Wolf's (1988) list of problems at the state level include "no consistency with regard to groups covered, definitions, mandatory reporting, investigation procedures, penalties, immunity, confidentiality and services" (p. 12).

Although this legislation has an important protective function, it may also lead to more guardianship cases. Guardianship results if a public agency required to investigate a report of abuse or neglect finds that the older person is uncooperative with the investigation, refuses to accept the services the agency recommends, rejects a recommended move to a nursing home, or opts to stay in an environment where he or she is being abused. If there are inadequate services available in the state to help the abused older person, then guardianship may be seen as the only alternative.

A number of programs around the United States can serve as models for elder abuse initiatives. In New York, Mt. Sinai Medical Center developed a comprehensive assessment and treatment program for abused elderly. Besides providing the treatment available in the hospital, the program helps abused older persons learn about their legal rights. The New Ventures program teaches volunteers to assist in managing finances and negotiating the health and human services system. In San Francisco, Community Agencies Serving the Elderly has developed a consortium of 55 community agencies that provide extensive services in cases of elder abuse (Models from Manhattan to Oahu, 1991). In Massachusetts, the Elderly Protection Program is a collaboration between local police departments and local adult protective service offices (U.S. Department of Justice, 1994). Under this program local police are provided background about issues in aging, financial exploitation of older persons, domestic violence, and other issues related to elder abuse. The National Center for Elder Abuse has provided grants to six communities to train professionals as "community sentinels." The community sentinels, including meals-on-wheels volunteers, are trained to spot signs of elder abuse and report these indications to local authorities. Over 1,000 community sentinels have been trained through this program (National Center on Elder Abuse, 2002).

REFERENCES

Administration on Aging. (1998). *Elder abuse prevention: What is elder abuse.* Retrieved from http://www.aoa.dhhs.gov/factsheets/abuse.html

Administration on Aging. (2001). *Elder rights.* Retrieved August 30, 2004, from http://www.aoa.gov/prof/aoaprog/elder_rights/LTCombudsman/National_a nd_State_Data/2001nors/2001OMBDS%20Reportfinal.pdf

Administration on Aging. (2004). *Fact sheets: Elder abuse prevention.* Retrieved August 30, 2004, from http://www.aoa/gov/press/fact/alpha/ fact_elder_abuse.asp

Ashville, N.C. Police Department. (2004). *Victims Assistance Unit.* Retrieved August 26, 2004, from http://www.ci/asheville.nc.us/police/cid/VIC-TIMS%20ASSISTANCE.htm

Barnett, H. (2004). Message from the president. *Legal Services Corporation, 2003–2004 annual report.* Retrieved November 28, 2005, from http:// www.lsc.gov/annualreport/0412101.pdf

Bigot, A., Demling, G., Shuman, S., & Schur, D. (1978). *Protective services for older people: A reanalysis of a controversial demonstration project.* Paper presented at the annual meeting of the Gerontological Society, Dallas, TX.

Blenkner, M., Bloom, M., Nielsen, M., & Weber, R. (1974). *Final report: Protective services for older people.* Cleveland, OH: Benjamin Rose Institute.

Blenkner, M., Bloom, M., Wasser, E., & Nielsen, M. (1971). Protective services for older people: Findings from the B.R.I. study. *Social Casework, 82,* 483–522.

Cantor, M., Brook, K., & Mellor, M. J. (1986). *Growing old in suburbia: The experience of the Jewish elderly in Mount Vernon.* New York: Fordham University Third Age Center.

Catalano, S. (2005). *National Crime Victimization Survey: Criminal Victimization, 2004.* Washington, DC: U.S. Department of Justice, Office of Justice Programs, National Institute of Justice. Retrieved October, 15, 2005, from http://www.ojp.usdoj.gov/bjs/pub/pdf/cv04.pdf

Horstman, P. (1977). Protective services for the elderly: The limits of pare IS patriae. In J. Weiss (Ed.), *Law of the elderly* (pp. 32–41). New York: Practicing Law Institute.

Kolasa, M., & Soto, M. (1990, October). *Legal hotlines to serve older people.* Paper presented at Third Annual Joint Conference on Law and Aging, Washington, DC.

Lake v. Cameron, 364 F. 2d 657 (N.C. Cir. 1966).

Legal Services Corporation. (2004). *Legal aid programs.* Retrieved August 27, 2004, from http://www.lcs.gov/welcome/wel_who.htm

Legal Services Developer. (n.d.). Oklahoma Department of Human Services, Aging Services Division. Retrieved August 26, 2004, from http:// www.okdhs.org/aging/legalservices.htm

Mathematica Policy Research. (1986). *National long-term care channeling demonstration: Final report.* Plainsboro, NJ: Author.

McEwen, T. (1995). *Victim assistance programs: Whom they serve, what they cf-fer.* Washington, DC: U.S. Department of Justice, National Institute of Justice.

Models from Manhattan to Oahu. (1991). *Aging Today, 12,* 15.

NARCEA Exchange. (1990). *Legislation and policy notes.* [Brochure] Wilmington, DE: Author.

National Center on Elder Abuse. (1999). *Types of elder abuse in domestic settings.* Retrieved August 30, 2004, from http://www.elderabusecente-/org/pdf/basics/fact1.pdf

National Center on Elder Abuse. (2002). *Sentinels: Reaching hidden victims.* Retrieved August 30, 2004, from http://www.elderabusecenter.org/pdf/sertinel/0205/pdf

National Crime Prevention Council. (2004). *Strategy: Crime prevention services for the elderly.* Retrieved August 27, 2004, from http://www.ncpc.org/ncpc/ncpc/?pg=2088-9598

National Senior Citizens Law Center. (2004). *About NSCLC.* Retrieved August 27, 2004, from http://www.nsclc.org/about_nsclc_programs.html

Office of the Inspector General. (n.d.). *State ombudsman data: Nursing home complaints.* Retrieved August 30, 2004, from http://www.oig.hhs.gov/oei-09-02-00160.pdf

Porter, D., & Affeldt, D. (1990). Legal services delivery systems: An overview of the present and a look at the future. In P. Powers & K. Klingensmith (Eds.), *Aging and the law: Looking into the next century* (pp. 89–112). Washington, DC: Public Policy Institute, American Association of Retired Persons.

Regan, J., & Springer, G. (1977). *Protective service for the elderly: A working paper prepared for the U.S. Senate Select Committee on Aging.* Washington, DC: U.S. Government Printing Office.

Schmidt, W., Miller, K., Bell, W., & New, B. (1981). *Public guardianship and the elderly.* Cambridge, MA: Ballinger.

Senior Victim Assistance Program. (2004). Retrieved August 26, 2004, from http://www.ctelderlyservices.state.ct.os/images/elderright.pdf

The triad solution: Alone no more. Retrieved August 26, 2004, from http://www.lapdonline.org/pdf_file/bsc/senior_citizens.pdf

Tomz, J., & McGill, S. (1997). *Serving crime victims and witnesses* (2nd ed.). Washington, DC: U.S. Department of Justice, Office of Justice Programs, National Institute of Justice.

U.S. Department of Justice. (1994). *National Crime Victimization Survey: Some findings from the Bureau of Justice Statistics: Elderly crime victims.* Washington, DC: Author.

U.S. Department of Justice. (2000). *Our aging population: Promoting empowerment, preventing victimization, and implementing coordinated interventions.* Retrieved August 24, 2004, from http://www.ojp.usdoj.gov/doc/ncj_186265.pdf

U.S. Department of Justice, Bureau of Justice Statistics. (2002). *Crime and victim statistics.* Retrieved August 27, 2004, from http://www.ojp.usdoj.gov/bjs/cvict_v.htm#summary

U.S. Department of Justice, Bureau of Justic Statistics. (2005a). *Crime and victim statistics.*Retrieved November 25, 2005, from http://www.ojp.usdoj.gov/bjs/cvict_v.htm#age

U.S. Department of Justice, Bureau of Justice Statistics. (2005b). *Violent crime rates declined since 1994, reaching the lowest level ever recorded in 2004.* Retrieved November 26, 2005, from http://www.ojp.usdoj/gov/bjs/glance/viort/htm

U.S. Department of Justice, Office for Victims of Crime. (2004). *Victim compensation and victim assistance.* Retrieved August 27, 2004, from http://www.ojp.usdoj.gov/ovc/publications/factshts/compandassist/fs_000306.htm#2

U.S. Senate Special Committee on Aging. (2000). *Elder fraud and abuse: New challenges in the digital economy. Hearing before the Special Committee on Aging of the U.S. Senate.* March 16. Washington, DC: U.S. Government Printing Office.

U.S. Senate Special Committee on Aging. (2003). *Guardianship over the elderly: Security provided or freedoms denied.* February 11. Washington, DC: U.S. Government Printing Office.

Wasser, E. (1974). Protective service: Casework with older people. *Social Casework, 97,* 103–114.

Wolf, R. (1988). The evolution of policy: A 10-year retrospective. *Public Welfare, 46,* 7–14.

CHAPTER NINE

Employment, Volunteer, and Educational Programs

For many elderly, retirement is a long-awaited event that promises to allow them to engage in long-postponed activities. It may also mean relief from the drudgery of a job that has been endured but never enjoyed. For other older workers, retirement is a dreaded moment, a termination of a career with its attendant status, a loss of important collegial relationships, and a future that promises to consist of hours of unfilled time. Activities for the elderly must therefore include both paid jobs and volunteer opportunities. Jack Ossofsky, former Executive Director of the National Council on the Aging, attempted to place the issue of employment and volunteer activities in a framework that transcends purely economic issues. "Maintaining options for the older American is the heart of the issue. . . . The greatest loss among the elderly is not economic status, income or health, serious as these may be. It's the loss of options, the opportunity to stay employed, volunteer for social work, start a second career" (Cattani, 1977, p. 13).

In this chapter we will examine both paid employment programs and volunteer opportunities available to the elderly.

EMPLOYMENT LEGISLATION

Age and Retirement

In 1900, two-thirds of men over 65 were still in the labor force. In fact, until 1950, over one-half of men over 65 were still working (National Council on the Aging, 1978). Whereas many workers elect early retirement, others feel forced out of jobs without any consideration being given to their experience and competency. National surveys indicate a mixed picture of retirement patterns: "Most older workers retire earlier than they had previously expected; however, nearly half work for pay at some point after retirement" (Moen, Erickson, Agarwal, Fields, and Todd, 2000, p. 5).

Until 2000, Social Security regulations placed some restrictions on the work options of the elderly as benefits have been reduced in proportion to earned income for people aged 65–69. Social Security limitations on earned income of workers who have reached the Social Security–designated full retirement age have now been removed. This change allows individuals to make a decision about their employment future knowing that they will retain their full benefits, regardless of whether they continue to work or retire. Some individuals may decide to continue to work or even seek new jobs because they enjoy working. Others may feel the need to continue to work because their pensions and Social Security benefits are not adequate to meet their financial needs. Whatever the reasons, approximately 10% of all workers in 2004 were over the age of 60 (Market reports, 2004). Among the total population over the age of 65, 13% were in the labor force in 2002 (U.S. Census Bureau, 2002). In that same year, 4.5 million individuals over the age of 65 were seeking work, an increase of 50% since 1980 (Knechtel, 2004).

Age Discrimination Legislation

The major allies of the elderly in their effort to obtain employment have been the Age Discrimination Employment Act of 1967 (ADEA), which outlawed discrimination based on age unless age was a bona fide requirement of the job, and the Age Discrimination Act. Originally the provisions of the ADEA covered employees in private firms, public agencies, and labor organizations who were between 40 and 65. For the elderly, the most important changes in the ADEA took place in 1978. The 1978 amendments increased coverage of the act to individuals up to 70 years of age in private and nonfederal employment. Mandatory retirement for most federal employees was abolished. The 1986 amendments to the ADEA outlawed mandatory retirement at the age of 70. Regulations accompanying the passage of the 1978 amendments to the ADEA transferred the enforcement of the act from the Department of Labor to the Equal Employment Opportunities Commission. This shift brought the ADEA enforcement under the wing of the agency charged with overseeing all other anti-discrimination activities. The effectiveness of the anti-discrimination efforts will become increasingly important as it is estimated that the number of workers over the age of 55 will increase from 18 million in 2000 to 32 million in 2015 (Knechtel, 2004).

Age discrimination complaints seem to vary with the state of the economy. If employers are facing economic problems, they often try to replace older, more expensive workers with less expensive younger men and women. The relationship between the state of the economy and age discrimination complaints can be seen in the 41% increase in complaints that occurred between 1999 and 2002 (Harris, 2003).

EMPLOYMENT PROGRAMS

Obtaining part-time and full-time jobs requires well-coordinated placement services that match skills of the worker to possible positions. Efforts in this direction are under way. Much less common are efforts to retrain older workers for new positions, which require extensive new skills.

Counseling

The first stage of employment efforts in many areas entails helping older workers gain a better understanding of their skills. This type of counseling has been part of the programs of voluntary agencies in Cleveland and Baltimore since the middle 1960s (Health and Welfare Council, 1965; Occupational Planning Commission of the Welfare Federation of Cleveland, 1958).

The counseling clinics attempt to provide the worker with supportive assistance, foster the development of self-assurance, and help with occupational adjustment. Meeting these goals involves attempting to overcome some of the common problems found among older individuals interested in or needing to work. These may include poor motivation or poor work histories, a long lag period since their last job, and a lack of appropriate skills for a changing labor market. Added to these deficits may be physical or emotional problems. Once counseling has helped to overcome these problems and enabled workers to achieve a realistic understanding of their own work potential, adequate placement becomes critical.

Using a variety of federal and local funds, placement programs are operating in a number of states and localities. This number could easily be expanded. Many of these programs are funded through provisions of the OAA, but a number of the most well-developed programs predate AoA's funding for employment programs. In 1959, the Atlanta branch of the National Council of Jewish Women (Cattani, 1978) started a placement program for older workers.

Older Americans Act Employment

On a national scale, the largest provision of funds for the older worker stems from Title V of the OAA. Prior to the emphasis on employment in the OAA, Title X of the Public Works and Economic Development Act of 1965 provided some job opportunities for the elderly. This program, targeted for high-unemployment areas, made some funds available for older workers. By 1975, approximately 4,800 seniors had obtained employment under this funding mechanism (Braver and Bowers, 1977).

The original Title IX of the OAA authorization of 1975 was aimed at helping needy older persons obtain a higher income level. It was also hoped that employment would provide these workers with a renewed sense of involvement with the community while they acquired new skills or upgraded existing ones. The OAA amendments emphasize serving "the needs of minority, limited English-speaking, and Indian eligible individuals, and eligible individuals who have the greatest economic need, at least in proportion to their numbers in the State and take into consideration their rates of poverty and unemployment" [Sec. 502].

The OAA also saw older persons as resources able to provide communities with needed additional human services workers, especially to fill major gaps in providing services to the elderly. The Senior Community Service Employment Program (SCSEP) of Title V has been contracted by the Department of Labor to a number of major organizations. These include AARP, Experience Works, National Asian Pacific Center on Aging, National Association of Hispanic Elderly, National Caucus and Center on Black Aged, National Council on the Aging, National Indian Council on Aging, National Urban League, Senior Service America, the U.S. Forest Service, and individual states. In 1975, 22,440 slots were authorized under the program (U.S. Department of Labor, 1977), but this figure had risen to 100,000 by 2000 and the total budget to $440 million in 2001 (U.S. Department of Labor, 2001). The major share of these funds (75%) is used to pay the wages of the older workers hired through this program. The remainder is used for related activities including job training, counseling, and placement (U.S. General Accounting Office, 2003). Classes in computer literacy and advice on how to handle questions related to age when interviewing with an employer have been found to be useful for SCSEP participants.

The 10 national contractors receive 78% of the moneys and the states 22%. Individual states receive funds in accordance with the percentage of state residents over age 55 and the per capita income of the state. A major concern of the program is to avoid political problems that would result if SCSEP workers filled job classifications normally held by full-time employees and were seen as competitive with these workers (National Council of Senior Citizens, 1987).

The efforts of Experience Works provide good examples of SCSEP activities. In 2001–2002, Experience Works trained and placed 30,000 low-income (income less than 125% of poverty level) individuals over the age of 55 in a variety of nonprofit and public organization settings (Experience Works, 2004). In all SCSEP efforts, the older adult has been limited to a maximum of 1,300 hours of work per year, averaging 20–25 hours per week, and payment of either the federal or state minimum wages, whichever is higher.

The Job Partnership Training Act (JPTA) earmarked 3% of its funds for poorer workers over the age of 55. The Act provided training and re-medial education as well as counseling and job search assistance. The training and assistance were oriented to private businesses. In the 1989–1990 program year, over 38,000 older participants were served through the "set-aside." In 2000, JPTA was replaced by the Workforce Investment Act and the set-asides for older workers were discontinued (U.S. Department of Labor, 2001).

Meeting Employment Needs

SCSEP participants are primarily women (73%). The majority of pro-gram participants are over the age of 65 (62%) (U.S. General Accounting Office, 2003). A major issue for the SCSEP is the ability of participants to move from jobs that are subsidized through OAA funds to unsubsi-dized jobs. The unsubsidized target goal of the OAA is 20%. The ability of SCSEP workers to obtain unsubsidized jobs will vary with the econ-omy. In 2001, 38% of Experience Works SCSEP participants found per-manent jobs. Prominent among the job classifications were clerical assistants, customer service representatives, and care providers (Experience Works, 2004).

Despite an inability to overcome the problem of obtaining unsubsi-dized jobs, the self-esteem and well-being attested to by SCSEP partici-pants has been seen as a testimony to its importance. The demographic profile of the United States is shifting, and fewer younger workers are available. Increasing numbers of employers may soon move on their own volition to hire older workers to meet their labor force needs, and the U.S. General Accounting Office estimates a large unmet desire for employ-ment on the part of older workers. An interest in hiring older workers is in evidence among fast-food and retail outlets, and is expected to increase during the remainder of the century. Hirshorn and Hoyer's (1992) re-search confirms the interest of private sector firms (with more than 20 employees) in hiring retirees. Many older people may welcome the op-portunity to develop new skills and talents if the working conditions are not onerous and the employment opportunities are interesting. One in-novative example is the program developed by the Environmental Protection Agency (EPA) to recruit older workers for employment in EPA laboratories and regional offices. The positions range from clerical to technical and professional. The program is administered through six national aging organizations. Although the Senior Environmental Employment program provides salary and benefits, workers hired under this initiative are not considered federal employees (U.S. Environmental Protection Agency, 2004).

VOLUNTEER AND INTERGENERATIONAL PROGRAMS

There are numerous opportunities available to older people who wish to serve as volunteers. The emphasis on older persons as volunteers has increased as the pool of women outside the paid labor force has shrunk. Older persons are thus recruited to assist museums and community organizations as well as traditional volunteer organizations such as the Red Cross. In addition to these general voluntary efforts, there are a number of programs oriented specifically to recruiting older persons as volunteers. At the federal level, the most important efforts are those administered through the National Senior Volunteer Corps, a component of the Corporation for National and Community Service. The programs more directly oriented toward the older person include the Retired Senior Volunteers Program (RSVP), the Foster Grandparents Program, the Senior Companions Program, and the Service Corps of Retired Executives (SCORE).

RSVP

RSVP's roots can be traced to a pilot program developed by the Community Service Society of New York in 1965. This project attempted to enlist older adults in volunteer work in the community and make use of their neglected talents and experience. The planners of project SERVE (Serve and Enrich Retirement by Volunteer Experience) hoped that the involvement of the elderly in the program would provide them with a renewed sense of self-esteem and satisfaction while filling important gaps in community resources.

The present RSVP program continues this tradition. Programs are locally planned and sponsored. Local communities must also provide 10% of the costs of the projects for the first year, 20% the second year, and 30% for the third and each subsequent year. Individuals enrolled in RSVP work in "volunteer stations," which include courts, schools, libraries, nursing homes, children's day care centers, and hospitals. Volunteers in the program include a retired minister who operates a commissary cart at a local nursing home and a retired lawyer who works one day per week at an Indian community center providing legal advice. Many volunteers are reimbursed for transportation to and from their assignments and for out-of-pocket expenses. The programs also provide the volunteers with accident and liability insurance. In FY 2001 RSVP projects utilized 480,000,000 volunteers and served 65,000 local organizations (Corporation for National and Community Service, 2004a).

Foster Grandparents

The Foster Grandparents Program is designed to provide low-income elderly with important social experiences while they assist children who have special physical or psychosocial needs. "Foster Grandparents do not displace salaried staff, but complement staff care to special children with the love and personal concern essential to their well-being" (ACTION, 1979, p. 3). Foster Grandparents work 4 hours a day in a variety of settings including correctional facilities, pediatric wards of general hospitals, homes for the mentally retarded or emotionally disturbed, schools, and day care centers. Foster Grandparents receive a nontaxable stipend in compensation for their efforts, reimbursement for transportation and meals, and accident insurance. To participate in Foster Grandparents, the older person's income must be no greater than 125% of the federal poverty level. The recruitment and training of Foster Grandparents is the responsibility of the individual program. The local programs also provide the older individual with counseling and referrals on personal matters. In FY 2001, the Foster Grandparents Program budget enabled 30,000 volunteers to be recruited to work with approximately 275,000 children and teens around the country. Because of its emphasis on assisting poverty-level elderly, Foster Grandparents programs have been emphasized in low-income areas (Corporation for National and Community Service, 2004b).

Senior Companions

The Senior Companion Program, which was authorized in 1973, is modeled after the Foster Grandparents Program, except that its stress is on low-income elderly working with other elderly. "Senior Companions may provide services designed to help older persons receiving long-term care, deinstitutionalized persons from hospitals and nursing homes, and others with special needs for companionship" (ACTION, 1979). The main emphasis of the program is on chronically ill homebound elderly. The volunteers must agree to serve at least 20 hours per week and at least 10% of project funds must be obtained from non-federal sources. By FY 2001, over 61,000 elderly were being assisted by 15,500 Senior Companion volunteers (Corporation for National and Community Service, 2004c).

Legislation enacted in 1986 now makes it possible for older individuals who exceed the income limits of the Foster Grandparents or Senior Companion program to join the program under certain conditions (U.S. Senate, 1991).

SCORE

The fourth program for older Americans is the Service Corps of Retired Executives (SCORE). Sponsored by the Small Business Administration, SCORE places retired executives in small businesses such as groceries, restaurants, bakeries, pharmacies, and other organizations that can benefit from their managerial experience. In New Bern, North Carolina, a SCORE volunteer helped a restaurant owner improve his financial and managerial skills. In Wenatchee, Washington, a SCORE volunteer helped develop a business plan for a couple interested in purchasing a store. In 2004, almost 11,000 older persons belonged to 359 SCORE chapters. These members provided services in a variety of formats including one-time counseling sessions, follow-up counseling sessions, and workshops.

Besides these efforts, intergenerational programming is now being implemented under the auspices of numerous agencies. Some of this programming is based on the premise that younger as well as older people benefit from intergenerational contact. Some of the increase in intergenerational programming is also due to the difficulties community programs have in obtaining adequate funds to pay staff.

Intergenerational programs can utilize youth to assist older people, as in the service-learning efforts on college campuses undertaken by the National Council on the Aging in the early 1980s (Firman, Gelfand, & Merkel, 1983). A more common approach is the utilization of older adults in programs for children, as in the Foster Grandparents model. Many intergenerational programs involve the sharing of sites between a program geared to children and one oriented to older adults. In Van Nuys, California, a day care program for children aged 6 months to 5 years shares a site with an adult day care program that works with dementia patients. Every activity that takes place at this site involves some intergenerational activity (Intergenerational programs, 2004). A larger scale program, the OASIS Institute, involves older volunteers in tutoring children. Over 4,000 tutors in 21 cities have been active in assisting children in advancing their reading skills. Begun in 1982 in four cities, OASIS programs are now offered in 26 cities at a variety of sites, including shopping malls.

To be effective, these activities need to be carefully planned. Generations United, a national organization, helps to develop intergenerational efforts and evaluate their effectiveness. Generations United members include 100 national, state, and local organizations (Generations United, 2004).

In order to assist in the recruitment and recognition of volunteers, the 1992 OAA amendments permit Area Agencies to hire a volunteer services coordinator. If more than 50% of the AAAs in a state develop a volunteer services coordinator position, the State Office on Aging must also develop a volunteer coordinator position. A section in Title III also supports expanded intergenerational programs in schools. The intent of this authorization is to provide intergenerational school-based programs, oriented to students with limited capacity in English and at risk of leaving school, drug abuse, remaining illiterate, or living in poverty. At the same time, by locating intergenerational programs in schools, older persons can obtain access to school facilities such as libraries, gymnasiums, theaters, and cafeterias (*Congressional Record,* 1992).

Older people who volunteer as tax counselors can serve individuals of all ages. The AARP Tax Aide program works in 8,500 sites and provides tax advice for individuals at libraries, senior centers, and community centers. Nationwide, 32,000 volunteers are involved in this program each year. The aides provide assistance for almost 2 million people (AARP, 2004).

EDUCATIONAL PROGRAMS

Educational opportunities for seniors have increased as institutions of higher education have recognized the potential for having adults of all ages on campus and the need to move some of their programming into the community. As the cohort aged 18–24 decreases, the opportunities for adults to fill their places in the classroom become more apparent.

Community Colleges

Community colleges have become community educational centers, not only for people seeking Associate of Arts degrees, but also for individuals wanting to upgrade skills and explore new areas of learning. Responding to this interest, many colleges have developed extensive noncredit programs that are offered both at the college and at sites in the community. For example, reading, literature, history, and art classes are often taken into nursing homes, senior day care centers, and nutrition centers. Many of these noncredit programs, freed from semester structure, can be offered on a flexible time schedule. They are geared to the older person and often designed in conjunction with groups of seniors.

  Community colleges have also encouraged older persons to take courses on campus through tuition waivers, pre-campus counseling, and remedial supports. For example, Dundalk Community College in Maryland offers a full semester of orientation for older persons. During orientation, each department is visited, time is spent in the labs and with the faculty, and remedial materials are made available. The campus-based courses include some geared particularly toward the elderly, as well as regular offerings that can be taken for credit or audited. The tuition waiver can come either through the decision of the college itself or as part of a city, statewide, or country program of tuition waivers. Because of the unique nature of the community college, it has done more to encourage older persons to become involved in education than any other educational group.

College and University Programs

Universities and 4-year colleges have also expanded their participation in educational programming for older persons, most commonly through tuition and fee reductions or waivers. Universities have provided everything from a minimum reduction in fees for audit only to full waiver of tuition and fees for any course or program of study. This latter approach usually offers all courses, degrees, and recreational facilities without cost to any state resident aged 60 and over. The first 2 years of the program often offer a full range of courses with the strongest emphasis on languages. Evaluation of these programs is showing that seniors who participated in these programs integrated themselves into the overall student body and did not ask for any special orientation, group meetings, or activities at the time they enrolled or at any later time. The university programs also appear to be primarily attracting older adults with previous college experience.

  The extent to which a college or university can offer free programs is dependent upon the size and status of the institution. For large state universities, the effect of 300 tuition-free students on the overall class structure will be minimal. For a small college or university, 300 students could make a significant difference in the course offerings and the size of classes. It is partly for this reason that educational opportunities for older persons vary greatly.

Elderhostel

Elderhostel is a national educational program that is gaining in popularity among older persons and educational institutions. This program sponsors 1-week courses on college campuses during the summer months.

Elderhostelers interested in participating in the program stay in dormitories with other summer students on the particular college campus during the week of courses. The purpose of the program is to create opportunities for Elderhostelers to live with other students, participate in campus activities, and take courses from regular campus faculty. The courses, designed for the 1-week program, are similar to those that would be offered to full-time undergraduates during the school year, and may include an introduction to music or astronomy, special history courses, or the flora of New England. Three courses are offered in each of the 1-week segments. A campus can offer as many weeks as it wishes for Elderhostelers, depending on the resources available.

The Elderhostelers come from throughout the nation and can go from campus to campus across the country. Each Elderhosteler must pay his or her own transportation and for the course, room, and board; there are no additional charges for the program. By 2004, 10,000 Elderhostel programs were being offered in 90 countries (Osborne, 2005). The enthusiasm among seniors for Elderhostel should not be surprising. As the number of older adults with extensive educational backgrounds continues to grow, there will be more demands on their part for advanced educational opportunities.

A locally based program is offered through the College for Older Adults of the Southwest Virginia Higher Education Center, a partnership of eight educational institutions. The College offers a variety of 6-week courses for interested adults over the age of 50 at extremely low cost (Southwest Virginia Higher Education Center, 2004).

Another set of innovative educational program for older persons is offered through the non-profit OASIS Institute. The emphasis has been on the humanities and wellness. Recent efforts have been focused on increasing Internet competency among older persons (OASIS Institute, 2003).

REFERENCES

AARP. (2004). *Hawaii: AARP tax aide needs your kokua.* Retrieved September 5, 2004, from http://www.aarp.org/states/hi/Articles/a2004-08-24-hi-tax-aide.html

ACTION. (1979). *Senior Companions Program history.* Washington, DC: Author.

Braver, R., & Bowers, L. (1977). *The impact of employment programs on the older worker and the service delivery system: Benefits derived and provided.* Washington, DC: Foundation for Applied Research.

Cattani, R. (1977, January 9). The elderly: Fight for job rights. *Christian Science Monitor,* pp. 12–13.

Cattani, R. (1978, January 11). Government job programs provide limited help to elderly. *Christian Science Monitor,* p. 15.

Congressional Record. (1992, September 22). Older Americans Act, Part II, H8969–H9006.

Corporation for National and Community Service. (2004a). *About Senior Corps: RSVP.* Retrieved September 8, 2004, from http://www.seniorcorps.org/joining/rsvp/

Corporation for National and Community Service. (2004b). *About Senior Corps: Foster grandparents.* Retrieved September 8, 2004, from http://www.seniorcorps.org/joining/fgp/index.html

Corporation for National and Community Service. (2004c). *About Senior Corps: Senior companion program.* Retrieved September 8, 2004, from http://www.seniorcorps.org/joining/scp/index.html

Environmental Protection Agency. (n.d.). *Senior environmental employment program.* Retrieved January 8, 2005, from http://www.epa.gov/ohr/see/brochure

Experience Works. (2004). *Senior workforce solutions.* Retrieved July 12, 2004, from http://www.experienceworks.org/scsep.html

Firman, J., Gelfand, D., & Merkel, K. (1983). Students as resources to the aging network. *The Gerontologist, 23,* 185–191.

Generations United. (2004). Retrieved September 4, 2004, from http://www.gu.org/index.html

Harris, S. (2003). *Simple justice. AARP Life Style.* Retrieved September 5, 2004, from http://www.aarpmagazine.org/lifestyle/Articles/a2003-05-221-mag-justice_age.html

Health and Welfare Council. (1965). *Older workers project: A demonstration on the job training program for workers over 50.* Baltimore, MD: Author.

Hirshorn, B., & Hoyer, D. (1992). *The private sector employment of retirees: The organization experience.* Detroit, MI: Wayne State University Institute of Gerontology.

Intergenerational programs, 2004. (2004). Retrieved September 4, 2004, from http://www.amda.com/caring/august2002/intergenerational/htm

Knechtel, R. (2004). *Productive aging in the 21st century: Employment of seniors.* Retrieved September 5, 2004, from http://www.go360.com/go60work.htm

Market reports. (2004). The mature market: Seniors and baby boomers market. Retrieved September 5, 2004, from http://www.thematuremarket.com/senorstratic/dossiert.php?numtxt=2216&drb=5

Moen, C., Erickson, W., Agarwal, M., Fields, V., & Todd, L. (2000). *The Cornell retirement and well-being study: Final report.* Ithaca, NY: Bronfenbrenner Life Course Center, Cornell University.

National Council of Senior Citizens. (1987). *Senior aides: A unique federal program.* Washington, DC: Author.

National Council on the Aging. (1978). *Fact book on aging.* Washington, DC: Author.

OASIS Institute. (2003). *Explore the possibilities: OASIS 2003 annual report.* Retrieved September 4, 2004, from http://www.oasisnet.org/about/OASISAnnual Report2003.pdf

Occupational Planning Commission of the Welfare Federation of Cleveland. (1958). *Measuring up: A career clinic for older women workers.* Cleveland, OH: Author.

Osborne, L. (2005, February 18). Never too old to learn. *New York Times,* pp. D1, 4.

SCORE. (2004).*Explore SCORE.* Retrieved September 5, 2004, from http://www.score.org/explore_score.html

Southwest Virginia Higher Education Center. (2004). *Degree programs and courses.* Retrieved September 5, 2004, from http://www.swcenter.edu/pages/coa.asp

U.S. Census Bureau. (2002). *Employment 65+.* Retrieved September 5, 2004, from http://www.census.gov/population/socdemo/age/ppl-167/tab09.pdf

U.S. Department of Labor. (1977). *Age Discrimination in Employment Act of 1967.* Washington, DC: U.S. Government Printing Office.

U.S. Department of Labor. (2001). *Older Americans Act of 2000: Legislative changes to the Senior Community Services Employment Act.* Washington, DC: U.S. Government Printing Office.

U.S. Environmental Protection Agency. (2004). *Senior environmental employment program.* Retrieved September 7, 2004, from http://www.epa.gov/epahrist/see/brochure/backgr.htm

U.S. General Accounting Office. (2003). *Older workers: Employment assistance focuses on subsidized jobs and job search, but revised performance measures could improve access to other services.* Retrieved August 22, 2004, from http://www.doleta.gov/performance/guidance/gaoreports/d03350.pdf

U.S. Senate. (1991). *Developments in aging, 1990.* Washington, DC: U.S. Government Printing Office.

CHAPTER TEN

Nutrition Programs

The Elderly Nutrition Program was formally authorized under the 1973 amendments to the OAA and provides at least one hot meal a day, primarily in a congregate setting, for those age 60 and over. Originally criticized by some as a new version of the Depression soup kitchen, this has become the most popular and universally well received program of the Older Americans Act. Its success can be attributed, at least in part, to the fact that it provides a measurable service (the preparation and serving of a meal) in a setting that brings people together informally while integrating its efforts with other available services in the community.

The goals of the program identified in 1973 by the AoA illustrate its dual emphasis:

1. Improve the health of the elderly with the provision of regularly available, low-cost, nutritious meals, served largely in congregate settings, and, when feasible, to the homebound.
2. Increase the incentive of elderly persons to maintain social well-being by providing opportunities for social interaction and the satisfying use of leisure time.
3. Improve the capability of the elderly to prepare meals at home by providing auxiliary nutrition services, including nutrition and homemaker education, shopping assistance, and transportation to markets.
4. Increase the incentive of the elderly to maintain good health and independent living by providing counseling and information and referral to other social and rehabilitative services.
5. Assure that those elderly most in need, primarily the low-income, minorities, and the isolated, can and do participate in nutrition services by providing an extensive and personalized outreach program and transportation service.
6. Stimulate minority elderly interest in nutrition services by assuring that operation of the projects reflects cultural pluralism in both the meal and supportive service components.

7. Assure that Title VII (changed to Part C under Title III in 1978) program participants have access to a comprehensive and coordinated system of services by encouraging administration coordination between nutrition projects and Area Agencies on Aging (AAAs). (Cain, 1977)

The first two goals also provide a summary of the success of the program. Nutrition is essential to good health but is greatly affected by the social situation. Eating is a social activity, and regardless of other resources, the older person is less likely to prepare adequate meals when eating alone. The last goal was strengthened in the 1978 OAA, which brought the administration of the nutrition program under the direction of the AAAs for the first time. Before 1978, the formal links with the AAAs were optional.

THE CONGREGATE NUTRITION PROGRAM

History

There have been conflicting data on the nutritional deficiencies of older Americans, based largely on the differences in urban, rural, ethnic, and economic variables. However, some general patterns of deficiency have emerged. "Calcium appears as the most common denominator, noted as deficient in most of the studies cited. Iron and Vitamins A and C are the next most commonly identified deficiencies . . . within the elderly, the problems of nutrition intake increase as the individuals grow older and are based as much in quantitative dietary shortcomings as in qualitative deficiencies" (Rawson, Weinberg, Herold, & Holtz, 1978, p. 27).

The malnourished elderly have been a part of our society for a long time, but formal, sustained programs to provide for those who do not have personal or financial resources are relatively new. The most significant research prior to the planning and development of a national nutritional program was the 1965 National Study on Food Consumption and Dietary Level sponsored by the Department of Agriculture. This study showed that 95 million Americans did not consume an adequate diet; 35 million of these had incomes at or below the poverty level. Subsequent analysis indicated that 6–8 million of those age 60 and over had deficient diets. These data laid the foundation for a federal nutrition program for the aged (Cain, 1977).

A task force set up to develop recommendations based on the results of the national study recommended demonstration projects for a 3-year period to determine the best mechanisms for delivering nutritional services. Demonstration projects were needed because of the lack of information on how such programs should be designed and, more important, the extent of their effectiveness (Bechill & Wolgamot, 1972). The purpose of the demonstration projects was to "design appropriate ways for the delivery of food services which enable older persons to enjoy adequate palatable meals that supply essential nutrients needed to maintain good health . . . in settings conducive to eating and social interaction with peers" (Cain, 1977, p. 142).

Although this overall goal seems straightforward, the demonstrations were expected to examine multiple issues. Besides the major effort to improve the diet of older adults, the meals were to be served in social settings that would allow for the testing of the effects of different types of sites. These sites would be evaluated in terms of their ability to promote increased interaction among the older clients. The effects of a nutrition education program on the eating habits of the elderly would be evaluated as well as the general ability of the congregate meals approach to reduce the isolation of older persons. Of course, the AoA was also concerned about the comparative costs of different methods of preparing and delivering meals and the problems that were entailed in any effort to increase the nutritional quality of the older person's diet (Cain, 1977).

The AoA funded 32 demonstration and research projects under Title IV. An intensive evaluation of the demonstrations produced the support for the national nutrition program first authorized in the 1973 OAA Amendments. The 32 demonstration projects were designed to control for variations in income, living conditions, ethnic background, environmental setting, staffing, and record keeping. This intricate design allowed national guidelines to be developed that would incorporate the successful components of each project. More important, the Title IV projects indicated to the AoA and the U.S. Congress that the proper provision of congregate meals for groups of elderly people fostered social interaction, facilitated the delivery of supportive services, and met emotional needs while improving nutrition.

It is clear that the risk of malnutrition among older persons has not been totally met. Older women and Black women were found in 2002 to be at higher risk of malnutrition than other groups of older persons (Sharkey and Schoenberg, 2002).

Program Operation

Under the provisions of the OAA, the AoA is mandated to develop a nutrition program for older adults

1. which, five or more days a week, provides at least one hot or other appropriate meal per day and any additional meals which

the recipient of a grant or contract may elect to provide, each of
which assures a minimum of one-third of the daily recommended
dietary allowances as established by the Food and Nutrition
Board of the National Academy of Sciences . . .

2. which shall be provided in congregate settings; and
3. which may include nutrition education services and other appropriate nutrition services for older individuals (Title III, Part C).

The nutrition program was developed at the federal level under the
authorization of the AoA and administered through a single agency. The
guidelines for operation have thus been clearer than in other programs,
such as home-delivered meals, which have developed out of different local and national program units.

Each state is allotted funds in proportion to the number of older persons in the state as compared with the older population nationally.
However, each state is guaranteed a minimum of .5% of the national appropriation. The federal government pays 90% of the cost of establishing
and operating nutrition services. The nutrition program is administered
by the state agency on aging, unless another agency is designated by the
governor and approved by the Secretary of the Department of Health and
Human Services. Based on a previously approved state nutrition plan, the
moneys are allocated to AAAs or public and nonprofit agencies, institutions, and organizations for the actual provision and delivery of meals.
Before the 1978 amendments, one-half of the local nutrition programs
were under the sponsorship of the AAAs, the other half under local sponsorship. Within 2 years of the 1978 amendments, all nutrition programs
were to be administered through the local AAAs to ensure service delivery coordination. However, AAAs are authorized to contract the nutrition programs to other local groups as appropriate.

The state units on aging and local nutrition administrative units must
provide for advisory assistance that includes consumers of the service at
the state level, members of minority groups, and persons knowledgeable
in the provision of nutrition services. Nutrition advisory groups can ad-
vise on all aspects of the program as well as play an advocacy role for its
continuation and growth. Programming, allocations, recruitment of participants, meal sites, and service linkage are common areas of concern for
nutrition advisory committees.

All persons age 60 and over and their spouses are eligible for services
under the nutrition program. Special emphasis is placed on serving the
low-income and disadvantaged elderly. This is achieved by locating nutrition centers, when possible, in areas that have a high proportion of
low-income elderly. Through this system, any variation of a means test is
avoided, thus increasing the general acceptability of the program to the

elderly, who often avoid programs that appear to be "charity." Actual centers or sites are located in any space appropriate for the serving of congregate meals. The centers can serve as few as 5 or as many as 250 participants on a given day; however, the average center serves between 20 and 60 participants each day.

Church basements, schools, high-rise apartments, senior centers, and multipurpose centers are the most common locations for nutrition sites. Because transportation is so important to the success of the program, centers are usually located in high-density areas where walking is possible, or on bus or subway lines. In suburban and rural areas, the centers are located in areas where some form of transportation to and from the center can be provided by the site. Unless the nutrition program is incorporated into senior centers that offer all-day programming, nutrition sites or centers are open up to 4 hours a day. The location of the center, available transportation, and additional resources affect the length of time of the daily operation of the program. For example, programs held in school cafeterias are often sandwiched between student lunch programs. In Illinois, lunches are served at 625 sites around the state. In Fiscal 2002, 46,000 meals were served at congregate sites (Illinois Department on Aging, n.d.).

Location also affects the type of programming developed by the site. Sites that are not used for other purposes allow greater freedom for alterations, decorating, and storage space than do locations that have other activities scheduled in the same space. Shared space has posed a hardship for many nutrition programs in meeting the national guidelines for program development.

The meals themselves are either prepared on site, delivered to the site in bulk, or delivered to the site in individual trays or containers. Because of cost and health code regulations, the on-site preparation is the least popular form of meal preparation. Catering services contracting with many nutrition sites in a given area can provide 6- to 8-week-cycle menus that both meet the nutritional requirements of the program and are interesting to the participants. Private firms, hospitals, and long-term care institutions are the most likely sources for meals because they can incorporate special diets into the program and already have an understanding of the nutritional needs of older persons. School cafeterias and restaurants are less successful meal sources. Catered meals arriving in individual trays provide the most flexibility for nutrition center locations, as health code requirements are minimal.

Eating and Socializing

Because the purpose of the nutrition program is to provide both meals and socializing, programming is an important part of the services offered.

When the nutrition site is incorporated into a high-rise for the elderly a senior center, or a recreation center, programming is usually part of the additional available resources. When the nutrition site is its own center, programming responsibility rests with the nutrition site managers under the direction of the nutrition project director for the region.

Programming is diverse and related to the interests and backgrounds of the participants. The programming available is similar to that found in senior centers, but with special emphasis on nutrition education, meal preparation, buying practices, health maintenance, and physical fitness. Not all participants become involved in the programming. Nutrition screening, assessment, education, and counseling are, however, basic components of the program.

Eating and Needs

People who attend the nutrition centers very often have other service needs. Because of this, the nutrition program has had to reach out and develop linkage with other community services. The nutrition programs have not built a duplicate service system but have, instead, integrated other agency services into their programs. Visits by Social Security representatives, health department officials, and recreation leaders are part of nutrition programming.

The limit on service funds has also been a factor in the location of nutrition sites. Many times, priority is given to sites located in existing community programs. For example, the nutrition program has led to the expansion of the multipurpose senior center system and has made possible many geriatric day care programs. County departments of recreation have been able to expand their programming because of the available lunch program. Housing developments for the elderly have also been able to build around the lunches being served.

Unfortunately, federal funding for both congregate and home-delivered meals has remained stagnant between FY 2002 and FY 2004. Funding limitations have necessitated links to other programs to fulfill the mandates of nutrition programs. Project directors have reached to other programs to supplement nutrition center staffing needs and have, in some cases, used senior aides and RSVP volunteers to provide support staff. Guidelines indicate that staffing preference should be given to older persons. In locations where the nutrition center or site is separate from other services, the staff usually consists of one part-time site manager assisted by volunteers. In this manner, the participants themselves become involved in the actual operation of the program, and see it as "their program" for which they feel responsible.

Funding

Funding for the basics of this program came from the federal government, with an initial outlay of $98 million. In 1975 and 1976, the amount was raised to $125 million and has continued to grow dramatically since then. The nutrition program is now the largest single component in AoA funding. In 2002, the Elderly Nutrition Program provided 108.3 million meals to almost 2 million older persons at congregate meal sites (National Council on the Aging, n.d.). Over $386 million was appropriated by Congress for congregate meals in FY 2004 (National Council on the Aging). Even with this funding, 40% of congregate meal providers have waiting lists of people who need this program (National Council on the Aging). To help compensate for these funding limitations, some sites require reservations, advance notice of cancellations, and in some cases, a 3- or 4-day rotating system of attendance. All of these requirements create hardships for older persons who have become dependent on these programs for an adequate diet.

Participants are encouraged to contribute something for the meal. The guidelines provide that individuals, from their own consciences, should determine how much they should and can afford to pay. Nutrition centers furnish envelopes or have similar systems in which participants pay what they feel is appropriate. The 1984 OAA amendments forbid programs from charging for their meals. Voluntary contributions, however, account for about 20% of the costs of congregate and home-delivered meals. Some congregate nutrition programs have adopted the use of posters to encourage older people to contribute for their meals. Others, such as the Columbus County Office for the Aging in New York State, have a suggested contribution scale. State offices on aging also receive surplus commodities or cash to supplement the cost of the meals they provide. The funding provided by the Department of Agriculture is based on the number of meals served with Title III funds. With the limited funding in some local areas in relation to the participant demand, participants have decided among themselves to contribute higher amounts so that more people can be served. Local donations and volunteers also help to defray about 14% of the costs of this program.

HOME-DELIVERED MEALS

Home-delivered meals ("Meals on Wheels") are provided to homebound persons and enable those who cannot buy food or prepare their own meals to have good nutritional meals on a regular basis. Approximately 90% of all those receiving homebound meals are aged 60 and over. The purpose of the program is to provide either one or two meals per day, 5 days a week. These delivered meals may enable many of these aged to remain living in the community.

History

Programs of home-delivered meals began in England immediately following World War II. The first program in the United States began in Philadelphia in 1955. The longest continuously operating program is "Meals on Wheels" of Central Maryland, Inc., which began in 1960 in Baltimore and was modeled after the English programs.

The early models of home-delivered meal programs were operated locally and largely by volunteer organizations. Originating in a church kitchen, these programs would serve from 15 to 100 clients, generating payment from clients either through a fixed fee or on a sliding scale. From 30 to 300 volunteers would be involved in any given local program. Referrals would come from friends, families, professionals in the field, or the elderly themselves. The number of daily meals and the costs of these meals both depended on the facilities available for meal preparation. Menus, number of meals served, amount, and cost were determined by the local organization sponsoring the program. Volunteers were primarily retirees and nonworking women, each of whom volunteered approximately 2 hours a week. The hot meal was delivered at noontime, and if a second meal was provided, it was a cold evening meal delivered at the same time as the hot meal. The early programs were sponsored by local churches, community groups, or nonprofit organizations and were largely self-sufficient, based on the fees charged the participating clients.

In the early 1970s, government funds resulted in either new programs under government sponsorship or links between nonprofit local programs and government agencies. With the introduction of these new support mechanisms, uniform standards, quality control, and uniformity began. The 1978 amendments to the OAA for the first time designated a separate authorization for home-delivered meals. This program was to be administered through the nutrition program. In some situations, there were no preexisting home-delivered meal programs. AoA-funded home-delivered meal programs primarily served clients who were congregate-site participants, whereas locally funded programs served other eligible clients. Because congregate nutrition participants often pay only when they feel they can, whereas those being served by a locally self-supporting home-delivered meal program pay a fixed fee, the Meals on Wheels cost to a client is often as much as five times higher. This can cause confusion when a client moves from one program to the other.

The 1978 legislation with separate authorization for home-delivered meals brought this issue of privately operated, largely volunteer groups vis-à-vis federally sponsored programs to a head. The authorizing legislation stated that home-delivered meal programs under the separate authorization were to be administered through the federal nutrition program, with preference for funding given to local preexisting voluntary home-delivered meal programs. Since 1978, OAA funding for home-delivered meals has grown dramatically.

Program Operation

In a home-delivered meal program, two volunteers—one acting as a driver, one as a visitor—visit 8 to 10 different clients each day. The volunteers spend 5 minutes with each client while delivering the meal. The home-delivered meal program's primary function is to prepare and deliver the meals, but it also provides a few minutes of friendly visiting. If additional services are needed, the client is referred to other support systems.

The meals are prepared by volunteers in church kitchens or are catered by private services, hospitals, long-term care institutions, schools, or colleges. When catered, the meals are either packaged by volunteers (delivered in bulk) or packaged by the meal-producing agency. The extent to which special-diet meals are available is determined by the amount of funds available and the source of the meal preparation. Low-salt and diabetic diets are the more common special diets available. The development of better serving boxes for keeping food warm and better individualized food-storage containers has improved the system of food delivery. Appropriate delivery equipment is essential to keeping the food at the right temperature without spoilage. Either a 6- or 8-week menu cycle ensures the variety necessary in such a program, while guaranteeing that the one-third required daily nutritional allowance is met in each meal.

When the home-delivered program is attached directly to the nutrition congregate site, the nutrition participants themselves often package and deliver the meals. In this way, those who are attending can keep in touch with participants who are unable to attend. As was pointed out in Congressional testimony (Cain, 1977), the longer the congregate nutrition program is available, the greater is the potential for home-delivered meals as part of the program. One project found that after 3 years, up to 30% of the participants were receiving home-delivered meals because of changes in their physical condition. The interrelation of the two programs is important so that those who are eligible for the nutrition program can continue, even when physical limitations temporarily make visiting the center impossible. The home program can speed recovery and perhaps, in many situations, make a return to the congregate site possible.

The 1978 amendments allowed individuals under 60 years of age to utilize AoA services. Because home-delivered meal programs have served anyone homebound, this legislation allows the younger homebound to continue to be eligible.

Funding

Nationally, the actual cost per day for the one hot meal and one cold meal delivered through the Meals on Wheels programs averages around $5 per meal. Funding to cover these costs has always been diverse. Either a fixed fee based on the cost of the meal, or a sliding scale that averages the cost of the meal has been the common method. In Skokie, Illinois, recipients of home-delivered meals pay $3.45 for a hot meal and $2.65 for a cold meal (Skokie, Illinois, n.d.). Recently, eligible clients have been able to use food stamps in most locations to supplement the cost of the meals. Currently, the $180 million in funds from Title III of the OAA (in FY 2004) are the key sources for revenue. These funds can be used not only for the cost of the meals themselves, but to pay those who prepare, package, and deliver them. Because of the availability of federal funds, there is a shift from volunteer to paid help for meal preparation and delivery. Local United Way, church, community service, and neighborhood groups also contribute money, equipment, or transportation to the program. Overall, funds from Title III enabled almost 2 million elderly to receive home-delivered meals (National Council on the Aging, n.d.). An additional number of home-delivered meals are provided through Title VI. Unfortunately, it remains difficult for many programs to provide home-delivered meals on weekends or holidays (Lieberman, n.d.).

It is clear that the elderly participating in nutrition programs have some major needs and that these programs are helping to meet some of those needs. Between 80% and 90% of nutrition program participants have incomes less than 200% of the federal poverty level, and are also twice as likely to live alone as other elderly. Possibly related to this social situation is the fact that two-thirds of these participants are either under- or overweight and have twice as many physical problems as other age peers (Administration on Aging, 1996).

Despite the growth of nutrition programs, it is clear that there will be increased demand for meal services, particularly among individuals over the age of 85 and the home-bound. Earlier hospital discharges will also result in many older persons being at home but unable to prepare the meals they need for proper convalescence.

REFERENCES

Administration on Aging. (1996). *Serving elderly at risk: The Older Americans Act nutrition programs: National evaluation of the Elderly Nutrition Program, 1993–95.* Washington, DC: Author.

Bechill, W. B., & Wolgamot, I. (1972). *Nutrition for the elderly: The program highlights of research and development nutrition projects funded under Title IV of the Older Americans Act of 1965, June 1968, and June 1971.* Washington, DC: U.S. Government Printing Office.

Cain, L. (1977). Evaluative research and nutrition programs for the elderly. In *Evaluative research on social programs for the elderly* (pp. 32–48). Washington, DC: U.S. Government Printing Office.

Illinois Department on Aging. (n.d.). *Nutrition programs.* Retrieved December 20, 2005, from http://www.state.il.us/aging/1athome/nutrition.htm

Lieberman, T. (n.d.). *Hunger watch: America's elders are waiting for food.* Retrieved January 8, 2005, from http://www.asaging.org/at/at-201/hunger.html

National Council on the Aging. (n.d.). Older Americans Act Appropriatons—Nutrition Services. Retrieved January 8, 2005, from http://www.ncoa.org/content.cfm?sectionID=165&detail=71

Rawson, I., Weinberg J., Herold, J., & Holtz, J. (1978). Nutrition of rural elderly in southwestern Pennsylvania. *Gerontologist, 18,* 24–29.

Sharkey, J., & Schoenberg, N. (2002). Variations in nutritional risk among Black and White women who receive home delivered meals. *Journal of Women and Aging, 14,* 99–110.

Skokie, Illinois. (n.d.). *Human services.* Retrieved January 8, 2005, from http://www.skokie.org/human/faqs.html

PART IV

Services for the Aged

In contrast to programs, existing services in aging offer a large number of components and always seem to be under pressure to expand. Because these services are community based, expansionist pressures often come from seniors in the community and their families.

This part will examine some complicated and vital service delivery systems, including multipurpose senior centers, housing services, in-home services, adult day care centers, and nursing homes. These services are presented in this chapter in a sequence that relates to their orientation to elderly with differing levels of need. Multipurpose senior centers serve ambulatory elderly, whereas housing services may be oriented to ambulatory elderly with some housekeeping and personal needs for which they require assistance. In-home services and adult day care centers serve seniors with more extensive physical or emotional problems. Finally, nursing homes are oriented toward a population that cannot survive in the community, even with the provision of extensive services.

It should be noted that although these services are discussed here individually, they are not mutually exclusive. Seniors may be taking advantage of more than one service. Ambulatory elderly who attend a senior center may also be living in elderly housing and receiving some home-maker assistance. Clients of adult day care centers may also be recipients of extensive in-home services.

Because of the variety of funding sources and varying eligibility standards, programs around the country have attempted to combine various sources of money with other local resources in order to be able to provide as broad a base of service as possible. In many areas this has blossomed into full-scale case management programs. The National Advisory Committee on Long-Term Care defines case management as:

a service that links and coordinates assistance from both paid providers and unpaid help of family and friends to enable elderly or disabled individuals with chronic functional and/or cognitive limitations to obtain the highest level of independence consistent with the capacity and their preferences for care. [Quinn, 1995, p. 8]

The committee has also defined six core functions of case management:

1. comprehensive assessment of the older person
2. development of a care plan based on the assessment
3. implementation and coordination of the care plan
4. monitoring of consumer and provider services to ensure their appropriateness and quality
5. comprehensive reassessment as needed
6. discharge from case management

In some communities, some of the needed services may not be available locally, creating problems for the case managers. As appropriate "packages" of services become more evident around the country, there has been increased effort to expand programs to enable case management to be effective in keeping the older individual in the community.

In Maryland, the Senior Care program serves moderately and severely health-impaired persons over 65 and attempts to help them maintain their residence in the community. Comprehensive assessment of the older individual and assignment of a case manager to help coordinate services are the basic components of the program. Limited "gap filling" funds are available when other programs are not sufficient to meet the older client's needs. The program is means-tested. A 1999 evaluation of the program by clients indicated a high level of satisfaction with the quantity and quality of services provided by Senior Care. Asked how they would cope without Senior Care, 50% of the users who participated in the survey indicated that they could manage living at home with support from friends and family members. The remaining 50% responded that they would have to move to a nursing home or assisted living facility (Maryland Department of Aging, 1999).

The Triage experience in Connecticut indicates that a well-conducted case-management approach can diminish the cost of providing services by reducing inappropriate institutionalization of the older person and the use of inappropriate community-based services. As a federally funded demonstration, Triage was allowed to waive some Medicare requirements for clients. Triage cost estimates were well below those of long-term residential care (Quinn, Segal, Raisz, & Johnson, 1982).

In many areas, case managers have no ability to affect the quality of a service except by refusing to refer individuals to a particular agency. Case-management programs in Monroe County, New York, and in San Francisco employ an approach that enables them to control the quality of programs they utilize. In Monroe County, the ACCESS program controls funds for the purchase of services. The On Lok program in San Francisco became well-known in the 1980s because of the comprehensive services it offers its clients. The PACE program described in Chapter 6 is an outgrowth of this effort not only to provide case management but also to actually provide the services that the older client needs.

Case management can also be an integral part of other programs, such as adult day care. In one national survey (Weissert et al., 1989), 79% of the day care centers under the auspices of general hospitals and social service agencies offered case-management services.

Case-management and supportive services may be even more crucial where family members live at a distance from their older relatives. The Jewish Family and Children's Agencies around the country have developed an Elder Support Network. Family members are able to arrange for case management and supportive services to be provided to their relatives living throughout the United States. The services are provided through local Jewish Family and Children's Agencies. Charges are on a sliding scale based on the family member's income. Similar services are available through networks of private social workers.

REFERENCES

Maryland Department of Aging. (1999). *Consumer satisfaction and effectiveness of the Senior Care system in Maryland*. Retrieved September 13, 2004, from http://www.mdoa/state.md/us/Services/scsurvey.pdf

Quinn, J. (1995). LTC case management: What it is and where it's going. *Aging Today, 26,* 7–8.

Quinn, J., Segal, J., Raisz, H., & Johnson, C. (1982). *Coordinating community services for the elderly: The triage experience.* New York: Springer Publishing Company.

Weissert, W., Elston, J., Bolda, E., Cready, L., Zelman, W., Sloane, P., et al. (1989). Models of adult day care: Findings from a national survey. *The Gerontologist, 29,* 640–649.

CHAPTER ELEVEN

Multipurpose Senior Centers

The multipurpose senior center is probably the most diversified service now available to the elderly. This diversity is emphasized in the National Council on the Aging's (NCOA) definition of a senior center: "a community focal point on aging where older persons as individuals or in groups come together for services and activities which enhance their dignity, support their independence and encourage their involvement in and with the community" (National Council on the Aging, 1979, p. 15).

This definition emphasizes the senior center as a community focal point, the key ingredient of present senior center philosophy. Senior center programs operate from a separate facility, serve as a resource for information and training, and promote the development of new approaches to servicing the older adult.

The OAA emphasizes the multipurpose senior center's role as a community facility for the organization and provision of a broad spectrum of services for the older person. The success of senior centers, however, lies not only in the breadth of services they provide, but also in the voluntary participation of the users in center activities. Seniors can choose not only whether they want to participate in a center program, but also in what way they want to become involved. Individuals thus maintain their independence while reaching out to others and to the community in a variety of activities.

HISTORY AND LEGISLATION

Associations of peers have always been sources of support for individuals. Clubs organized for older people can be traced as far back as 1870. However, centers for older people began with a program in New York City in 1943. The idea came from workers in the New York City Welfare

Department who felt that the older people with whom they were working needed more than a club. The organizers of the project, besides securing a meeting place, had contributed games, had suggested the serving of refreshments to foster sociability, and, having gathered the old people together, expected that they could manage by themselves. In this way they had provided them with a more sociable means of passing time, which then seemed adequate provision. No one had thought beyond this point (Maxwell, 1962).

The idea of this form of association quickly spread, as private groups began setting up centers throughout the country. The San Francisco Senior Center, begun in 1947, was created through efforts of the United Community Fund, the American Woman's Volunteer Services, the Recreation Department, and individual local citizens (Kent, 1978). In 1949 the new "Little House" in suburban Menlo Park, California, was able to attract while-collar and professional clients (Maxwell, 1962).

Senior centers grew primarily as locally supported and directed institutions. Established either by local nonprofit groups or by local units of government (departments of social service or departments of recreation), centers were designed to be primarily responsive to local needs. However, most of the growth in senior centers has occurred since 1965. Before that time, small clubs were the most common form of social organization. Even in 1970, there were only 1,200 centers, as opposed to 10,000 in the 1990s (Krout, 1995).

In the 1970s, federal legislation made more funds available for the development of senior centers. The most important piece of authorizing legislation was Title V of the OAA. The 1973 amendments, Section 501, inserted into the act the new "Multipurpose Senior Centers" title. Although not funded until 1975, this title identified senior centers as a unique and separate program. Because Title V provided funds for "acquisition, alteration, or renovation" of centers, but not for construction or operation of centers, Title III made it possible to fund senior centers for the development and delivery of a variety of specific services. Title V provided resources for the facilities, and Title III provided operational monies.

The 1978 amendments to the OAA consolidated the Title V program into Title III, repealing Title V. With this change, Title III can "provide for acquisition, alteration, renovation, or construction of facilities for multiple purpose senior centers as well as provide for the operations of these centers." This consolidation provides for a greater opportunity to organize senior centers under the direction of the AAAs. The new Title III also allows the AAAs to fund senior centers from their beginning to fully operational stages.

A number of other legislative enactments provide mandates for senior centers.

1. The local Public Works Development and Investment Act of 1965 provided funds that may be used for the development of multipurpose senior center facilities. Under Title I of this act, funds may cover 100% of the cost of construction, renovation, and repair of buildings to be used as centers.

2. The Social Services Block Grant, Title XX of the Social Security Act, provided funds for group services for older persons in senior centers. Many of the programs offered through these centers were eligible for funds under this title, because Title XX's purpose was the provision of social services for low-income persons. Only individuals who met the eligibility requirements could receive services. Because of this requirement, it was often difficult to coordinate the Social Services Block Grant programs with those funded through the OAA, which had no eligibility requirements other than the age of the recipient.

3. The Housing and Community Development Act of 1974 provides funds for the expansion of community services, principally for persons of low and moderate income. Construction funds are available through this act (Administration on Aging, 1977).

CHARACTERISTICS

Senior Center Users

By 2003, there were an estimated 12,000 senior centers in operation across the United States (Aday, 2003). A survey of senior centers in seven states found an average age of 75 among users. On average, the participants had attended the centers for 8.3 years (Aday). In 1984, senior center participants represented 15% of the population over age 65. The attendance at senior centers represents a usage rate 4 to 12 times greater than that of any other community-based programs for older persons.

There has been a strong interest in differentiating users from nonusers of senior centers. Krout's 1988 review of research on this issue did not provide any definitive answers. The variables that did not differentiate users from nonusers of senior centers include sex, age, marital status, degree of loneliness, and lack of transportation.

Studies of the effects of race and ethnicity on senior center usage have produced mixed findings, as have variables including occupation, income, educational differences, health status, and degree of social contact with others. Whereas these reported studies were based on local samples, an analysis of national data (Krout, Cutler, & Coward, 1990) found a number of important factors related to senior center participation. These included "higher levels of social interaction, lower income, increasing age up to 85, living alone, fewer ADL and IADL difficulties, higher education up to post–high school, being female, and living in central city or rural nonfarm areas" (p. 79). Miner, Logan, and Spitze (1993) attempted to clarify the determinants of attendance by analyzing data from the 1984 Supplement on Aging to the National Health Interview Survey. They found that individuals who participate and use senior centers most frequently are poorer, more socially active, and older. The age variable is complex in its effects, as after a certain age, individuals are less likely to attend a senior center. Neither race, subjective health status, nor frequency of usage was found to determine center attendance. There was also no relationship between functional disability and frequency of usage, although the most disabled individuals are less likely to participate in senior center activities.

Although race was not a predictor of senior center usage, participation of African American and Latino elderly in senior centers has been low. A survey of 424 senior centers (Krout, 1994) found that 24% had an increased number of non-White participants. Ralston and Griggs (1985) found a significantly higher commitment to senior center programs among African Americans than among Whites. Although African Americans may have more difficulty getting to the centers, African American women were more encouraged by children to attend the senior center than were White women. As the numbers of minority elderly increase, there is a need for more senior centers oriented to these populations. In New York City, Latino elderly are estimated to comprise 20% of the older population. Based on these numbers, there should be approximately 68 senior centers dedicated to serving the Latino population. In 2002, there were only 16 (Latino Gerontological Center, 2002).

Models

The early centers in New York and Menlo Park became the prototypes for the two conceptual models of the senior center that are now dominant. One conceptual approach embodied in the social agency model views senior centers as "programs designed to meet the needs of the elderly and postulates that the poor and the disengaged are the more likely candidates for participation in senior centers." The alternative "voluntary organization model hypothesizes that the elderly who are more active in voluntary organizations and who manifest strong attachments to the community are also the ones who make use of senior centers" (Taietz, 1976, p. 219).

Early research identified the social agency model as the most commonly developed. As Taietz notes, the social clubs for the elderly have been most meaningful to individuals who are isolated from social relationships, helping to relieve their loneliness. For the older person who is active in a number of informal and organizational roles, the existence of age-graded social clubs may not seem an exciting opportunity.

The voluntary organizations are usually groups that have many social activities but also have regular memberships and organizational by-laws, and conduct scheduled meetings of the members on a variety of topics (Taietz, 1976). In a study of senior centers in 34 communities, Taietz noted the similarities between senior centers and other voluntary organizations that include both service components and professional staff. One major difference, however, was that, whereas veterans and fraternal groups tend to be sex-exclusive, senior centers provide men and women with equal access to programs. However, because the centers under this model are similar to formal voluntary organizations, their major clientele will tend to be active elderly rather than more isolated seniors.

In an exploratory study, Sabin (1993) found support for both models, with different types of programs and clientele patronizing the respective programs. Whereas centers that utilized the social agency model had more of an emphasis on services, centers oriented to the voluntary agency model had more focus on self-expression, recreation, and collective action. These centers were more attractive to higher-income and more active older persons.

Fowler (1974) proposed three different criteria for categorizing senior centers. The first defines centers in terms of activities generated. The center can be identified by whether it primarily provides services, activities, individual services and casework, or a combination of the three. The second mechanism for categorizing centers is by administration. The center administrative core may be centralized (everything in a central facility), decentralized (located in several neighborhood facilities), combined (central location, with satellites), or a multiplicity of operations with some linkage. Finally, centers can be classified by the origin of their services. The services can be offered exclusively by center staff, by center staff and community agencies, or by community agencies with the center staff providing coordination. The descriptions of the models themselves show how complex and diversified the structure can be and still come under the rubric of "senior centers."

As part of the National Council on the Aging (1979) study of centers, another model emerged, one based on size and complexity of operation and including four levels:

1. Multipurpose senior center
2. Senior center
3. Club for older persons
4. Program for all persons, with special activities available for elderly

The differences between centers and clubs do not rest solely in their activities or membership, but rather in the breadth of services available to clients, the permanent nature of the physical facility, and the numbers of unpaid staff. Many senior centers are also incorporated entities.

Cohen (1972) attempted to further differentiate the center from the club. The center was viewed as having the following five characteristics:

1. Community visibility based on a good facility and easy identification
2. A central location for services, through either a central site or satellites
3. An ability to serve as a focal point for concerns and interests
4. An ability to serve as a bridge to the community
5. A program purpose that focuses on the individual, family, and community

The diversity of structure, size, and functioning capabilities is a result of the origins of senior centers. The centers have emerged from the community; are sponsored primarily by voluntary, nonprofit, or public community-based organizations; and still receive a substantial percentage of funding from locally determined sources.

PROGRAMMING

Although center programming is diverse, it falls into two basic types: recreation-education and service. The programming provided is most likely to be successful when it is built as part of the larger community structure and under the direction, or at least with the support, of the older people who will be served by the center.

Recreation and Education

Recreation-education is the type of programming most commonly conceived as the central component of a senior center. It is this that sets it apart from other service delivery agencies in the community, and builds the center as a neighborhood focal point for seniors.

The development of activity and the selection of the activities to be offered are related to the target group identified by the center. If the center plans to serve everyone within a given geographic area, the programming should reflect the diversity of the population served. Whether clients are men or women, people of high or low income, people of various ethnic backgrounds, or from urban or rural settings should be reflected in the activities designed for the center. If not, unrepresented components of the population potentially served will not utilize the center because their activity needs are not being met. Taietz (1976) warned program directors of the danger of neglecting the special efforts required to attract isolated and alienated elderly to the centers. Hanssen and colleagues (1978) added another cautionary note with the identification of another subgroup for whom activity programming is not always available:

> The senior center does not consistently accommodate those seniors with perceived physical limitations and those who are mildly depressed. This finding highlights a critical problem for senior centers. If they are to provide services beyond recreation, they must help those persons with greater perceived health problems and that have other limitations. [p. 198]

This early caution about services for frail elderly has continued to attract attention, as senior center directors note that more of their clients appear to be frail. Although 58% of the senior centers reported an increase in frail elderly in Krout's (1995) survey, this increase may represent not only the attendance of new individuals, but also the aging in place of long-standing members. Accurate tallying of the numbers of frail elderly receiving services at senior centers is difficult because of the lack of clear definition of the term "frail."

Many senior centers make special efforts to serve elderly with special needs. These elderly may have serious chronic illnesses and physical impairments. It is clear, however, that resources, adequately trained staff, and attitudes toward the frail elderly are among the problems faced by centers interested in serving this important population of older persons (Krout, 1995). With increased emphasis in federal programs on the "frail elderly," we can expect these programs to expand.

The recreation-education component of center programming can be as varied as the community resources allow and as the participants' interests indicate. Common activities include arts and crafts, nature, science and outdoor life, drama, physical activity, music, dance, table games, special social activities, literary activities, excursions, hobby or special interest groupings, speakers, lectures, movies, forums, round tables, and community service projects. When center participants themselves identify their interests and plan the activities with expert assistance from staff, there is a greater chance of adequate participation and success.

Services

The services component of programming is the other essential ingredient for a successful senior center. What identifies the senior center as the community focal point for older people is the combination of activity and service in one location. The availability of a lecture on horticulture, dental screening, or square dance lessons, along with Social Security advice at the same site and with the same friends, makes the senior center a unique community resource.

The services available through a senior center depend on the facilities, the resources, and the community supports available. These services can be provided directly by center staff, by agency staff assigned to the center, through satellite centers close to the agency, or by the agencies themselves rotating through the center.

Services likely to be available through senior centers fall into a number of categories (Cohen, 1972).

1. Information, counseling, and referral, including general information; intake and registration; personal counseling; referral resource files; and special group education around special problems.
2. Housing and living arrangements and employment, including helping the older person locate appropriate housing situations; job referral and counseling programs; and job retraining.
3. Health programs, including screening clinics for a variety of health problems; pharmaceutical services; specialty services, such as dentistry, podiatry, hearing, and speech; and health education programs. These programs are most likely to be developed in conjunction with county health departments, doctors, nurses, extended-care facilities, hospitals, and outpatient clinics in the area.
4. Protective services, including preventive services such as planning for the appropriate use of funds or securing safe living arrangements; supportive services to help enable the older person to be as self-sufficient as possible; and intervention services, including assistance in gaining access to such legal resources as commitment or guardianship.
5. Meals, such as those provided through the OAA nutrition program. The development of the nutrition program since 1973 has been the single biggest contributor to the development of senior centers. Because the nutrition program needed sites for the congregate meals and senior centers needed a meal program in order to continue adequate daily programming, the nutrition program has given the centers a much-needed resource.
6. Legal and income counseling, including help in determining eligibility for Supplemental Security Income (SSI) and the preparation of wills.
7. Friendly visiting as an outreach program, with the participants of the center providing the visiting and outreach services.
8. Homemaker assistance.

9. Telephone reassurance and buddy programs.
10. Handyman and fix-it programs.
11. Day care services.
12. Transportation programs.
13. Nursing home resident activities within the senior center facility.

This list, developed in the 1970s, was still pertinent into the 2000s. The most common efforts reported by 424 centers were information and referral, transportation, and congregate meals (90%). Home-delivered meals were provided by 70% of the centers (Krout, 1995).

The majority of self-identified multipurpose centers offer at least educational, recreational, and either information and referral or counseling services. Many multipurpose centers also provide health services and opportunities for volunteers.

It is clear that effective programming is essential for a senior center to fulfill its role as a community focal point. Because senior center participants are more likely to attend by choice, or at least see their first coming to the center as motivated by choice rather than need, relevant programming determines the continued attendance of older community residents.

Programming Examples

Perhaps the best way to gain an overview of the multipurpose senior center is to examine some examples of centers that illustrate the wide range of programs that can be offered in these facilities.

The senior center in Franklin County, New York, is run under the auspices of the county's office on aging. Because the office serves a rural population, the primary service of the eight senior centers is transportation: 12- and 20-passenger vehicles provide 9,000 rides a year to the center, stores, and health facilities. In addition, the center provides full-time nutrition, education, physical fitness, and craft programs. Assistance is also provided to seniors who are applying for special government programs. In the smaller communities in the county, senior citizen clubs meet monthly for social purposes. The clubs' membership links up with the senior centers for trips and other cooperative events.

The Waxter Center in Baltimore provides one of the most comprehensive services in the country. Built as a result of a $4 million bond issue, the center now has over 11,000 members. Housed in a large, specially designed three-story building, Waxter offers a range of activities including swimming, language classes, crafts, a library, lectures, and trips. Because a large number of separate rooms are available, 15 to 20 different activities can be carried out at the same time, giving each member a wide choice of individual or group settings. The center also operates an extensive health screening clinic, an adult day care program, and a special program to integrate nursing home patients with center members. Representatives from Social Security, SSI, Legal Aid, home care agencies, and other public agencies are at the center on a daily basis. The center, including the nutrition program, is open 7 days a week.

The Hudson Guild-Fulton Senior Center in New York City has a membership of 1,300, with 300 members present on any given day. An advisory committee helps to make decisions affecting the staffing operations of the center and to initiate programs that respond to their own interests and talents. The center views itself as a supermarket, with members selecting what they need from its offerings. The center's classes include crafts, exercise, drama, music, discussions, and languages. Tickets are available through the center to the wide range of concerts, theater, and opera offerings that are available in New York throughout the year.

The Hudson Guild-Fulton center provides assistance to its members for Medicaid, Medicare, Social Security, and other public-assistance problems. Personal and housing problems, as well as legal concerns, also receive attention from the center staff and volunteers. Clients are assisted in finding jobs and volunteer placements. Health-screening programs and a telephone reassurance program help to maintain the health of the elderly and keep them in contact with the center. A minibus transports members to health care appointments. The center also provides breakfast to about 30 seniors and lunch to an average of 200 older adults at the center and to 75 in their homes.

Although this description of senior centers concentrates on concrete services, the center also has an important role in maintaining the self-esteem and integration of the older person in the society (Gelfand & Gelfand, 1982). Intergenerational programming can help to break down age segregation, and membership in the center can help foster identity of older persons with an organization at a time when their organizational affiliations are diminishing.

The center can also provide an opportunity for older individuals to develop new roles that may have been stymied by the demands of their daily work patterns. Perhaps most important of all is the opportunity for older persons to develop friendships. These friendships may result from the general socializing that they engage in at the center. Indeed, there are indications that it is this opportunity for socializing, rather than specific programs, that attracts many older people initially to senior centers (Gelfand, Bechill, & Chester, 1989; Ralston, 1987). These opportunities to socialize may, in turn, lead to the enlargement of the older person's support network. The new members of the network may become confidants. In some centers, "quasi-formal" support groups have developed among members who are friends and keep tabs on important events in each other's lives. When some negative event occurs, such as the loss of a spouse or family member, they help by sending cards or visiting and gradually bring the person back into center activities.

Senior centers can also provide support to family members, including those who are caregivers to older relatives. This support may be simply educational in nature, or it may take the form of groups that allow the caregivers to share feelings and problems. The center can be viewed not merely as a service-delivery operation, but as a facility that has the potential to meet some of the important emotional and social needs of the older person. Use of this perspective can make a major difference in the attitudes and programming of the staff.

The importance of the senior center for many participants should not be underestimated. In Aday's (2003) seven-state study, 75% of the respondents said that senior center programming helped them remain independent. An even larger proportion (90%) reported that they developed friendships at the center and 50% relied on friends from the senior center for assistance. In addition, 87% felt that their friends at the senior center provided them important emotional support.

Senior centers need to attract the "young-old" as participants or the median ages of the participants will continue to rise and senior centers will be characterized as programs that exclusively focus on the frail elderly. The effort to attract younger seniors is already producing an emphasis on programs such as fitness and exercise. In Chicago, the Department of Aging has initiated free fitness and strength and training class at its senior centers (*Health and Medicine Week*, 2004). Senior centers thus need to avoid being characterized as facilities with programs that exclusively focus on the frail elderly and have an ability to attract "baby boomers." Senior centers will have to adapt to the life style of this cohort of older individuals: "Many boomers will continue to work either full time or part time as they age. They're not going to come and spend the day at a senior center. Instead they'll pick, choose and pay for classes scheduled during evening and weekend hours at different sites including libraries and other community buildings" (Schneider, quoted in Vann, 2003). The ability to maintain a position not only as a multi-service provider, but as a provider for all diverse groups of older persons, is a major challenge for senior centers.

FACILITIES

Because senior centers can present an image that encourages older persons' participation in center programming, the choice of a facility has always been a very important part of senior center development. The fact that under the old Title V of the OAA monies were available only for the development of the center's physical plant underscores the importance of appropriate facilities: "A senior center should be a place in the community which is attractive and makes older people feel that it is a place where they want to come. In addition, an attractive facility represents to the community that older people are valued by both the community and themselves" (Administration on Aging, 1977, p. VI-1).

In order to maximize opportunities for securing a wide range of clients, attempts are always made to locate a senior center in an area convenient to transportation. This location should also be in a neighborhood that is accessible to the target population. Adequate parking facilities, outside activity spaces, and easy accessibility for the handicapped are also vital elements of the physical plan. The interior of the center should provide a variety of room sizes including private areas for counseling, a kitchen-dining area, and adequate space for staff and supplies.

A national study (Krout, 1990) indicated that three-quarters of senior centers were housed in separate facilities. Among centers that are combined with other types of settings, 33% were included as part of recreation/community centers, 20% in multiservice agencies, 12% in churches, 7% in housing facilities/projects, and 6% in schools. An additional 20% were housed in a variety of other settings.

With the rising costs of building, rehabilitating, and renovating facilities, it is anticipated that development of adequate facilities could continue to be a barrier to expanding the senior center programs. Fortunately, in many communities, unused schools have been changed to senior centers. The recycling of buildings that had related purposes can help keep down costs.

FUNDING

Funding mechanisms for senior centers reflect the importance of integrating the center into the community. There is rarely a single source of support for all the activities that a center may wish to inaugurate. Instead, funding from a variety of sources is utilized to cover different components of the center's activities.

The auspices under which the center is operated may thus be a crucial determinant of the sources of funds a center is able to tap.

A number of federal funding sources are available to centers including the following:

1. Title III of the OAA authorizes funds for multipurpose senior center construction, operation, nutrition services, and special programming. Title IV authorizes training and research funds as

well as model projects. Title V can fund senior community service employment programs through senior centers.

2. Block grants from the Department of Housing and Community Development can be utilized for developing, improving, and co-ordinating senior center activities and facilities.
3. As determined by the locality, General Revenue Sharing funds can be allocated to senior centers.
4. The volunteer programs of ACTION can provide additional personnel resources for the senior center.
5. If deemed a priority, a state may allocate funds from the Social Services block grant.
6. Funds from the Higher Education Act can assist centers in developing educational activities and for the training of center staff to implement a variety of learning projects.

In addition to federal funds, state and local monies are also available. Centers have been funded through legislative appropriations in many states, and several centers have been financed through a bond issue, either city- or state-supported. Civic and religious organizations often make contributions to senior centers. Because the center is visible, contributions by these groups not only provide needed resources to the centers, but bring some visibility to the contributing organization. These groups can most easily donate labor, space, materials, and equipment.

Private philanthropists and nonprofit groups also are likely to make contributions, and United Way, as well as local private foundations, can be a source of annual support. Finally, the center itself can generate some income from membership dues, fund-raising projects, or the sale of center-generated products.

Most centers attempt to combine funding from a variety of sources, with the primary source Title III of the OAA. However, significant support has been made available by the Department of Labor, state and county funds, state and local revenue sharing, in-kind contributions, United Fund, religious organizations, foundations, membership fees, civic groups, and project income. Because in-kind contributions account for a substantial amount of support, center budgets are difficult to estimate. Free space, volunteers, and service agency personnel are all important, but are hard to quantify in dollars-and-cents terms.

REFERENCES

Aday, R. (2003). *Identifying important linkages between successful aging and senior center participation.* National Council on the Aging/American Society on Aging Joint Conference, March 12–16. Retrieved September 13, 2004, from http://www.aoa.gov/prof/aging/net/Seniorcenters/NISC.pdf

Administration on Aging. (1977). *Program development handbook for state and area agencies on multipurpose senior centers.* Washington, DC: U.S Government Printing Office.

Cohen, M. (1972). *Senior centers: A focal point for delivery of services to older people.* Washington, DC: National Council on the Aging.

Fowler, T. (1974). *Alternatives to the single site center.* Washington, DC: National Council on the Aging.

Gelfand, D., Bechill, W., & Chester, R. (1989). *Maryland senior centers: Programs, services and linkages.* Baltimore: School of Social Work, University of Maryland.

Gelfand, D., & Gelfand, J. (1982). Senior centers and support networks. In D. Biegel & A. Naparstek (Eds.), *Community support systems and mental health* (pp. 162–174). New York: Springer.

Hanssen, A., Meima, N., Buckspan, L., Henderson, B., Helbig, T., & Zarit, S. (1978). Correlates of senior center participation. *Gerontologist, 18,* 193–199.

Health and Medicine Week. (2004, May 31). Geriatrics: Focus of senior centers shifts to fitness, p. 536. Atlanta, GA: Author.

Kent, D. (1978, May–June). The how and why of senior centers. *Aging, 281–282,* 2–6.

Krout, J. (1988). The frequency, duration and stability of senior center attendance. *Journal of Gerontological Social Work, 13,* 3–19.

Krout, J. (1990). *The organization, operation and programming of senior centers in America: A seven year follow-up.* Fredonia, NY: Unpublished.

Krout, J. (1994). Changes in senior center participant characteristics during the 1980s. *Journal of Gerontological Social Work, 22,* 41–55.

Krout, J. (1995). Senior centers and services for the frail elderly. *Journal of Aging and Social Policy, 7,* 59–76.

Krout, J., Cutler, S., & Coward, R. (1990). Correlates of senior center participation: A national analysis. *The Gerontologist, 30,* 72–79.

Latino Gerontological Center. (2002). *Older Hispanic-Americans left behind in the greatest need.* Retrieved September 13, 2004, from http://www.gero-latino.org/lead1.html

Maxwell, J. (1962). *Centers for older people.* Washington, DC: National Council on the Aging.

Miner, S., Logan, J., & Spitze, G. (1993). Predicting the frequency of senior center attendance. *The Gerontologist, 33,* 650–657.

National Council on the Aging. (1979). *Senior center standards: Guidelines for practice.* Washington, DC: Author.

Ralston, P. (1987). Senior center research: Policy from knowledge. In E. Borgatta & R. Montgomery (Eds.), *Critical issues in aging policy: Linking research and values* (pp. 199–234). Newbury Park, CA: Sage.

Ralston, P., & Griggs, M. (1985). Factors affecting utilization of senior centers: Race, sex, and socioeconomic differences. *Journal of Gerontological Social Work, 9,* 99–111.

Sabin, E. (1993). Frequency of senior center use: A preliminary test of two models of senior center participation. *Journal of Gerontological Social Work, 20,* 97–114.

Taietz, P. (1976). Two conceptual models of the senior center. *Journal of Gerontology, 31,* 219–222.

Vann, K. (2003, August 26). Senior centers anticipating arrival of hip boomers. *The Hartford Courant.* Retrieved April 21, 2004, from http://www.global-aging.org/rural_aging/us/centers.htm

CHAPTER TWELVE

Housing

HOUSING CONDITIONS OF THE ELDERLY

Housing is a crucial aspect of the social environment. The type and quality of housing available to older persons have an impact on their general level of satisfaction, and on their ability to live in the community. Retired older persons also spend more time in their homes than younger, working individuals. A few statistics help to clarify the housing situation of older persons:

- Over 1,000,000 older households (6%) live in housing that needs repair or even rehabilitation.
- Three-quarters of persons over the age of 65 own their own homes.
- More than 30% of all elderly households allocate over 30% of their income for housing costs.
- Among renters, approximately 900,000 spend more than 30% of their income on housing.
- Older residents of public housing are "poorer, older, and frailer than most elderly households" (U.S. Department of Housing and Urban Development, 1999).

In 1999, there were already 2.5 million households headed by a person over age 62 (AARP, 2001). A 1992 survey by AARP of those over the age of 55 found that 84% of the respondents wanted to stay in their current home and that only 6% were living in any form of housing developed for older adults. This 6% figure will probably grow as the older population continues to age and a greater variety of senior housing becomes available.

Many older individuals with limited incomes have taken advantage of the subsidized housing made available through the Department of

161

Housing and Urban Development or local state agencies. More affluent elderly have increasingly shown interest in retirement communities with specific age limits for residents or new continuing care ("life care") communities. There is also increasing evidence that many older persons who have no children or grandchildren living with them are interested in living in central cities where they have access to restaurants and cultural events: "I've been to around 40 cities in the last couple of years, and in every one of them there is either a small and growing or a very large movement back downtown. . . . There's no question it's a national phenomenon, it's happening even in Rust Belt cities, and it's fueled by groups: young professionals and empty nesters" (McIlwain, 2004, p. 4). In recognition of this trend, builders are planning retirement communities on the outskirts of cities such as Chicago.

This chapter discusses the major privately and publicly sponsored housing services available to the elderly. As the history and current program models indicate, there are two streams of funding, one that provides monies for the building of units for low-income families, and a second that subsidizes the costs of rentals for low-income families. Table 12.1 provides a list of the major federal housing programs available to older persons and the numbers of older people they serve.

History

The concept of federally supported housing began in the 1930s with the National Housing Act of 1934 and the United States Housing Act of 1937. The 1934 Act inaugurated the first home mortgage program—a restructuring of the private home financing system—under the Federal Housing Administration (FHA). Under the 1937 Act, the government offered subsidized housing to low-income families. Although the primary purpose of this latter legislation was to clear slums and increase employment, new housing resulted. Under the Housing Act of 1949, the national goal of "a decent home and suitable living environment for every American family" was first stated. The act also included programs for urban renewal, increased funds for subsidized housing, and new programs for rural housing. During the 1950s, housing programs were more directed toward rehabilitation, relocation, and renewal.

Section 202 began under the Housing Act of 1959. The program provided low-cost loans to developers of private housing and was the forerunner of later mortgage subsidy programs. In the Housing Act of 1961, below-market interest rate mortgages were initiated to assist rental housing for moderate-income families through section 221(d)(3). In 1965, two rent-subsidy programs were begun. In one program, residents would pay 25% of their income in privately owned housing units built

TABLE 12.1 Occupancy of Older Persons in Major Federal Housing Programs

	Program	Number of Older Persons
Targeted to older persons	Section 202 Supportive Housing for the Elderly	221,753
Targeted to older persons and disabled	Section 231 Mortgage Insurance for the Elderly	8,145
With special features for the elderly	Section 515 Rural Rental Housing Loans Housing Choice Vouchers	152,439
	Project-Based Rental Assistance (includes Section 8 and rent supplement in properties not included elsewhere in Table) (inactive)	330,475
	Public Housing	181,073
	Section 207/2233(f) Mortgage Insurance for Existing Multifamily Properties	288,094
	Section 221 d(3)(4) Mortgage Insurance	87,588
	Section 236 Mortgage Insurance and Interest Reduction Payments (inactive)	60,524
	TOTAL	1,362,192

Source: Government Accountability Office, 2005.

with FHA financing. Under the Section 23 leasing program, the government would lease regular units for low-income families.

In 1968, Congress found that "the supply of the nation's housing was not increasing rapidly enough to meet the national goal of 1949" (U.S. Department of Housing and Urban Development, 1973). Congress then established a production schedule of 26 million housing units—6 million of these to be for low- and moderate-income families over the next 10 years. One of the programs of this act was Section 236 which provided a subsidy formula for rental housing. In 1969, the Brooke Amendment was passed, which limited the amount of rent that could be charged by local housing authorities to 25% of adjusted tenant income.

In September 1973, President Nixon halted all housing programs except the low-rent public-leasing program, in order that a thorough review could be accomplished of what was then viewed as a spendthrift and inadequate program (U.S. Department of Housing and Urban Development, 1973). Following a study, during which no new federally subsidized housing starts were approved, the Housing and Community Development Act was signed into law in August 1974. The act removed the suspension that had been placed on construction and required contracts annually of at least $150 million to help finance development or acquisition costs of low-income housing projects. Because most of the money was to be channeled through the new Section 8 program, which was authorized under this Act, funding was slow to begin. Administratively, at least 2 years elapsed before the Section 8 program was fully operational (U.S. Senate, Special Committee on Aging, 1975).

Public Housing

Although the term is often assumed to relate to all forms of subsidized housing, "public housing" was in fact the earliest means of providing adequate homes for low-income elderly. Public housing was established under the Housing Act of 1937. The Department of Housing and Urban Development (HUD) appropriates funds for these complexes. More than 1 million households live in rental units administered by local housing authorities. The authorities maintain the buildings and ensure that low-cost rentals are available to poor families. Rentals are usually set at 30% of the family's income. In addition HUD provides funds for maintenance of the buildings, and other agencies may provide staff for special programs for older persons.

It is often difficult for older persons to live in public housing units because many local housing authorities require that older residents who need supportive services arrange to have these needs met if they are to remain in the complex. A small percentage of housing authorities (10%) do not allow older persons who are not independent to live in the public housing complex.

In 1999, 13% of public housing tenants were seniors (U.S. Department of Housing and Urban Development, 2000). Many of these tenants had aged in place. In recognition of the needs of this population, the National Affordable Housing Act of 1990 allows local housing authorities to charge HUD for the inception of "service coordinators" positions and for 15% of the cost of services to older tenants. These services may include meals, chore services, transportation, personal care, and health-related services. Approximately half of all public housing units are over 20 years old. In recent years, the federal emphasis in the field of housing has shifted to other programs such as Section 8 and Section 202.

The Section 8 Existing Housing Program

Authorized under the Housing and Community Development Act of 1974, this program filled the void left by the 1973 moratorium. It provides no direct funding to the developer, but instead pays monthly rent, so that housing can be developed on the private market.

Section 8, or subsidized rent, is the rent for a unit in a development receiving federally subsidized Section 8 housing assistance payments. The Section 8 rent differs from the market rent in that it depends strictly on the amount of income of the tenant. Tenants pay 30% of their adjusted income for rent, with the Section 8 housing assistance payment to the landlord making up the difference between tenant-paid rent and the full market rent (U.S. Department of Housing and Urban Development, 2004b). Tenants are now allowed to pay more than 30% of their income for rent if the public housing authority agrees that the rent is reasonable for both the unit and the family (U.S. Senate, Special Committee on Aging, 1991). The tenant could pay as little as $40 or $50 per month or nearly as high as the market rents, depending on the monthly adjusted income.

Rents under Section 8 cannot exceed the fair market rent for the area as established by HUD. Rents are reviewed annually, and the tenants must move if 30% of their adjusted income meets the fair market rent for that particular housing project. Fair market rents take into account construction costs and maintenance fees for individual locations. Tenants in housing built through Section 202 grants usually receive Section 8 subsidies.

Fair market rates vary widely. In Oakland, California, the fair market monthly rent for a one bedroom apartment is $1,132, in San Diego, $939, Atlanta, $815, and in Chicago, $797 (U.S. Department of Housing and Urban Development, 2004b).

In order to qualify for Section 8 subsidies originally, the income of a family of four could not be above 80% of median income in their area of residence. Congressional action between 1981 and 1984 reduced eligibility to 50% of median income, thus making many families ineligible for Section 8 subsidies. Nationally, families with less than 30% of the local median income comprise 75% of the families receiving subsidized rent (U.S. Department of Housing and Urban Development, 2004b).

Projects with Section 8 rental units are owned by private parties, profit and nonprofit, and by public housing agencies. Under Section 8, HUD has made 15- or 20-year contracts with private parties for the rental units, unless the project is owned by or financed with a loan or loan guarantee from a state or local housing agency. In this case HUD will guarantee the rental units for 40 years. Efforts have been made to increase the private guarantee time of 20 years because in some situations it is a disincentive for private parties to become involved in the program. Any type of financing may be used for the purchase or rehabilitation of a project that houses Section 8 rental units, including HUD-FHA mortgage insurance programs, conventional financing, or tax-exempt bonds.

The property owner handles the whole program and is responsible for leasing at least 30% of the subsidized units to eligible families. Under the Section 8 legislation, priority is given to projects with 20% of their units in Section 8 only to guarantee an income mix in the housing project. However, if the rental units are to be used for the elderly, there is no restriction on the number of Section 8 rental units per project. Older persons occupy approximately half of all Section 8 housing.

The purpose of the Section 8 program is to develop rental housing for very low-income families within the structure of the private housing market. Section 8 units can exist in houses, small apartment buildings, or any other location that has units to rent. Suburban, rural, and urban areas are equally eligible. However, HUD determines how many Section 8 rental units can be awarded to a given area in each state. Usually, applications far exceed the units available for the specific areas in question.

The Section 8 housing program had a slow beginning after it was authorized in 1974. In 1975, there were 200,000 applications, but only 30 new units actually materialized (U.S. House of Representatives, 1976). The cumbersome application and administrative procedures were blamed for the delay. Section 8 was an entirely new program involving low-income families. The private financial community—the group that had to generate the construction monies—did not appear ready to fund the building of units that would house Section 8 families until the program had grown to become one of the key housing programs for the elderly. Section 8 covers only the actual rental units, but is most successful when combined with other housing construction and service programs.

Concerns about cost appeared to create questions about the development of any large number of Section 8 units in the 1980s. By 1989, 46% of Section 8 housing was occupied by older persons. Section 8 rent subsidies are now available only for existing housing. Subsidies for new housing were eliminated in the Housing Act of 1983 (U.S. Senate, 1990).

The federal government planned to renew many of these for short terms. Funding for Section 8 housing had also declined from $293 million in FY 1996 to $128 million in FY 1997 but had returned to $249 million in FY 2004 (NAMI, 2004). As a possible alternative to the Section 8 Existing Housing Program, the Reagan administration instituted housing vouchers, which allow individuals to find their own housing in the private sector. In the voucher program, tenants also contribute 30% of their income to the rent. A payment standard based on fair market rents is determined for the local area. If the rent of the tenant's unit is less than the payment standard, the tenant's contribution is reduced by the difference. If the rent exceeds this payment standard, the tenant must make up the difference. There are no limits in the rent the tenant can pay under the housing voucher program (Leger & Kennedy, 1990). Housing vouchers have been authorized for only 5 years.

An evaluation of the experiences of a large number of enrollees indicates that the housing voucher program has been successful (Leger & Kennedy, 1990). Questions have been raised from the onset of the program as to whether enrollees will be able to find housing they can afford and landlords who will accept the vouchers. In areas with tight housing markets, these two factors could pose a major hurdle. The average success rate in 1990 for finding housing was 65%. There were, however, three areas with lower success rates, and one area where the success rate was only 33%. The reasons for these differences could not be clarified. Overall, housing voucher recipients were slightly more successful in obtaining qualified housing than were recipients in the existing housing certificate programs.

Over one-third of the recipients were able to stay in their existing apartments while obtaining vouchers. Housing voucher recipients who moved paid rents that were 6.7% higher than recipients in the certificate program. This difference may, in part, reflect "higher prices for higher quality units" (Leger & Kennedy, 1990, p. xii). Older persons had better success rates than younger age cohorts, and single-person older households had the highest success rate of any group. The success rate of older persons in the voucher program was somewhat higher than in the certificate program. There was a significant reduction in the rent burden of elderly in the voucher program. The elderly were the only population group for which a significant difference was found.

The Section 202 Program

Authorized under the Housing Act of 1959, Section 202 provides a capital advance at no interest to interested nonprofit organizations. The advances do not have to be repaid if the housing units remain available to low-income elderly for at least 40 years (*$5.2 billion,* 2003). The rents paid by tenants in Section 202 housing do not usually cover the costs of operating the property. To cover these costs, the program also provides rental assistance to the nonprofit organizations. Rental housing can be provided for the elderly through new construction or rehabilitation of existing structures. The property should include needed support services and can have such rooms as dining halls, community rooms, infirmaries, and other essential services. These supportive services are largely funded by funds from non-Housing and Urban Development sources. Many of the nonprofit homes for the aged, such as Cathedral Residences in Jacksonville, Florida—a large housing complex that serves over 700 elderly—were partially constructed with money under Section 202.

The Section 202 program was very successful throughout the 1960s, but was phased out after that time in preference to Section 236, another federal loan program. However, Section 236 was frozen in 1973 when all federal housing programs were halted to allow for review. Section 202 was reinstated as part of the Housing and Community Development Act of 1974, but it did not return to full activity until the summer of 1975. Under the 1974 act, a $215 million borrowing level was approved for FY 1975, but it was not used until the following year. Regulations in 1976 reaffirmed the importance of the program in providing both construction and long-term financing for housing projects (U.S. Senate, 1991). By 2003, 350,000 units had been funded through the 202 program. Typically 6,000 units of new housing are funded through the program each year (*$5.2 billion,* 2003). In fiscal 2002, $783 million was available for Section 202 programs. (U.S. General Accounting Office, 2003). In 2004, older persons constituted 85% of the households utilizing the Section 202 program (Government Accountability Office, 2005). Despite this impressive figure, only 8% of very low-income elderly renters were being helped by 202 housing (*$5.2 billion,* 2003).

Private nonprofit corporations and consumer cooperatives are eligible for Section 202 financing. Housing developments under Section 202 cannot exceed 300 units. Section 8 participation is required, and approval of Section 202 loans is based on the feasibility of getting Section 8 financing. In other words, Section 202 construction financing cannot be granted if the number of Section 8 units for a section of the state has already been obligated. Section 202/8 allocations are made in accordance with Section 213, a fair share needs formula. The formula, which determines the number of eligible units for a given geographic area, is based on the following criteria:

1. the number of households with the head or spouse age 62 or older,
2. the number of such households that lack one or more plumbing facilities,
3. the number of such households with incomes less than the regionally adjusted poverty level, and
4. the prototype production costs for public housing units as adjusted by average cost factors within the loan region.

The target population for Section 202 programs is an elderly household—one headed by an individual over the age of 62—with income less than 50% of the median income in an area. In 2003, approximately 3.3 rental households in the United States qualified under these income criteria (*$5.2 billion*, 2003). The 1974 Housing Act also specified that 20–25% of funds for Section 202 housing must be awarded in rural areas. The residents of the housing must also reflect the racial population of the community. This provision was meant to ensure that minority elderly obtained housing. The projects are required to have either an adequate range of necessary social services or to facilitate the access of residents to such services. The application process for Section 202/8 housing is extensive and consists of five stages. It usually takes 3 to 5 years from the time of idea to actual implementation, and approval is given only to those developers with a proven track record.

Although Section 202 projects continue to be built, the size of these projects has dropped substantially. Some of this reduction in size is related to the growth of 202 projects outside of central cities: 22% of the projects occupied after 1984 were built in areas with fewer than 10,000 residents, a figure that is in stark contrast to the 2.2% of the projects occupied before 1975. As in previous years, religious groups (50%) sponsor the largest proportion of projects. The 202 program provides 86,000 units for needy older persons around the country (*$5.2 billion*, 2003).

Other Federal Housing Initiatives

Section 231 insures lenders against losses on mortgages for construction or rehabilitation of unsubsidized housing for the elderly. This program is available to both profit and nonprofit developers. By FY 1989, 67,000 units of housing for older persons were insured under this program. Although not specifically targeted for the elderly, Sections 221(d)(3) and (4) play a larger role at present in insuring multifamily housing for the elderly. In 2002, 38,000 units with a value of $3 billion were insured through Section 221(d)(4) (Weichert, n.d.). These two sections permit the inclusion of congregate programs in the developments they insure. One of the innovations of 221(d)(4) was Retirement Service Centers, which provide rentals at the market rate for older persons but also include congregate meals, housekeeping, and laundry services. Although the program had completed 128 projects providing almost 19,000 units by 1990, it was suspended by the Department of Housing and Urban Development. The decision to suspend this program was based on a default rate in excess of 35%.

Section 223(f) provides mortgage insurance for existing multifamily housing units for the elderly where the repair needs are not extensive; this program is available in connection with refinancing or purchase of a project (U.S. Senate, Special Committee on Aging, 1990). Section 236 authorized interest-reduction payments on behalf of owners of rental housing projects designed for occupancy by lower-income families for the purpose of reducing rentals for such tenants. In recent years units built through 221(d)(3) and 236 financing have become unavailable to low-income tenants as landlords have prepaid their mortgages and raised the rents. The 1990 National Affordable Housing Act allowed landlords to sell the property. If a nonprofit group interested in purchasing the property cannot be found, the property can be sold. Older or disabled tenants, however, must be given 3 years to find another apartment. The displaced tenants will be given vouchers to subsidize their housing, and the former landlord will pay 50% of the moving costs (Retsinas & Retsinas, 1992).

The 1990 Housing Act also contained two important new initiatives. The HOME Investment Partnership provides block grants to localities with the expectation that most of these funds will be used for rental assistance, assistance to home buyers, or construction or rehabilitation of homes. The Home Ownership and Opportunity for People Everywhere (HOPE) reflects national support for an idea that originated with a public housing complex in Washington, D.C. HOPE provides funds that allow public housing tenants who would not receive mortgages from banks to purchase their units. HOPE is oriented to first-time homeowners. In the Seattle-Tacoma area in 1996, 10 homes were purchased by the local housing authority and rehabilitated. Families with an average income of $25,000 were selected for low-cost mortgages and allowed to purchase these newly renovated dwellings. The local community that receives HOME funds must match the federal grant. In 2001, 125,000 rental units had been completed with HOME funds and 16% of these units were occupied by individuals overs the age of 62 (AARP, 2001).

State and Local Housing Programs

State and local housing agencies have become an important source of financing for the actual building or rehabilitation of housing units. These agencies provide mortgage money directly to developers through sale of notes and bonds. Construction financing may be provided through the sale of notes, and permanent loan funds are provided through the sale of long-term bonds. The bonds sell at an interest rate of 1–2% below that of conventional sources of real estate financing. These low rates allow housing agencies to pass on the savings on the notes and bonds to developers in the form of lower interest rates, which result in lower rents and mortgage-carrying charges for market-rate tenants and home buyers.

The purpose of the housing agency programs is to attract private developers to the low- and moderate-income housing field with the aim of providing housing for a broad range of income levels. The programs usually place a limit on equity return to developers.

Services

The various HUD programs and state housing agencies support housing that ranges from public ownership and complete public financing to private financing, building, and renting, with federal insurance on the mortgage only. The upper-income limits allowed vary by program, with the most stringent limits placed on the direct public housing and the least stringent limits on the mortgage insurance-only program.

As indicated earlier, nonprofit developers are free to design as much additional space as they wish, and are encouraged to add supportive services to the housing units financed under Section 202. However, because of the income limitations placed on those living in federally financed housing, the developer has to keep the rents within the fair market rates and within the rates that the limited-income residents can pay. This, in turn, places limits on the amount of additional support services that can be provided. For example, one high-rise for the elderly in Baltimore, financed under Section 202/8, has the entire top floor overlooking the city as a carpeted and draped multipurpose room. The cost of building as well as maintaining this large, well-equipped, and well-used room must be absorbed in the rental fees allowed for each individual apartment. With the rental ceilings determined by the government, the room can be only marginally maintained.

Amenities built into the housing programs depend on available finances and on the cost of these amenities. The support from the community in maintaining additional housing facilities and regional preferences will also be determinants of a final design package. The potential resources that can be included in elderly housing are extensive, ranging from transportation, nutrition, and health-screening programs to craft rooms, groceries, and even small restaurants.

Elderly housing projects can thus be part of the larger service-delivery system of the community. Because federal housing funds are limited, services run under outside auspices may need to be incorporated into the housing units. Two excellent examples of housing complexes with integrated services are Worly Terrace, Columbus, and Glendale Terrace, Toledo, Ohio. Geared to the elderly who are returning from mental hospitals and to low-income community residents—many of whom were losing their homes through urban renewal—these housing developments operate a unique series of integrated financing and service systems. Whereas HUD paid for the basic construction of the units, the state of Ohio paid for the rooms not eligible under federal regulations (in this case, dining room, community building, clinic, and craft room); the local housing authorities manage the completed housing units.

Worly Terrace is located near public transportation, shops, and several churches. The complex has a six-story high-rise building with 106 living units, four one-story buildings with 120 units, and a centrally located community building. There are furnished and unfurnished quarters for as many as 270 residents, with apartments for single persons, couples, or two unrelated single persons to share. Available services include hot meals, beauty and barber services, preventive health services including health screening, services of a full-time registered nurse and licensed practical nurse, part-time physician and podiatrist, social activities, and recreation (U.S. House of Representatives, 1976). The services available in publicly financed or insured housing depend on the developer, the sponsor, the interest of the residents, and the community resources available. Early planning and community support for the project enhance the chances for adequate support services. Many states are using Medicaid waivers that allow them to utilize Medicaid funds for services in elderly housing sites. Case managers and home care workers may set up offices in individual buildings where a large proportion of the residents are older (Mollica, 2003).

Home Repair and Renovation

Many older homeowners find it necessary to seek alternative housing because of their inability to carry out the maintenance necessary to keep their homes in good condition. They also may lack the funds to hire contractors to perform necessary repairs. As homeowners quickly learn, minor repairs that are delayed for a substantial period of time can easily become major costly ones.

Home repair programs aimed primarily at low-income elderly have now been organized around the country. Many of these programs have dual purposes: (1) bringing substandard homes up to local code levels, and (2) providing supplemental income by hiring older persons to work on these projects.

In Evansville, Indiana, a major repair program for elderly residents was carried out in a number of neighborhoods. As in other geographic areas, the repair efforts were concentrated on functional aspects of the home including wiring, vermin control, replacement of broken window panes, and new plastering. The hope of the project coordinators was that instituting the repair program would produce a ripple effect, which would not only encourage the elderly to continue making their own repairs, but also encourage other neighborhood residents to undertake long-needed repairs. One of the reasons this ripple did not occur was because a majority of the elderly did not even tell their neighbors about the program. This silence was attributable to their ambivalent feelings about accepting aid. In order for the program to be more visible within the community, the evaluators argued that the repairs would have to be undertaken on a continuous basis, rather than bringing repairmen into the individual home for an intensive, but brief, period of time (Abshier, Davis, Jans, & Petranek, 1977).

Home repairs that are to be anything more than cosmetic are also costly, although volunteer labor can reduce costs significantly. In one community, a neighborhood corporation provides regular home repair and renovation services for over 2,000 enrollees (McCleary, 1986).) In Fiscal 2004, more than 1.5 million older persons received services through the Community Development Block Grant (U.S. Department of Housing and Urban Development, 2004a). Home repairs and rehabilitation were among the major uses of these CDBG funds by older recipients. Funding for home repairs can also be developed from a variety of possible sources including Title III of the OAA, the Social Services block grant, or local appropriations. In rural areas, low-interest home repair loans are available through the Farmers Home Administration Section 504 Program. Under the Department of Energy Weatherization Assistance Program, low-income elderly can also apply for funding to help them purchase energy-saving aids, such as storm windows or insulation.

Congregate and Assisted Housing

Housing for the elderly should respond to the wide variation in the needs of older persons. The growth in the interest and availability of assisted or congregate housing is a response to the need for housing among those elderly who cannot continue to maintain full independent living, and yet are not in need of some form of full-service institutional setting. In part, the increase in need for this type of housing is related to increased average longevity, a phenomenon in which a greater proportion of the total population is over 75 years of age and has conditions that require some forms of care in addition to basic housing needs.

Service needs in housing programs often increase as the tenants age. Tenants who entered the housing program as healthy, independent persons find they need additional service supports with advancing age. New, unanticipated services are then required. Congregate housing is an environment that provides enough services to enable many impaired elderly to remain in a community-based residential situation. Lawton (1976) focuses more precisely on the services that might be available in such a congregate housing situation: "Congregate refers to housing that offers a minimum service package that includes some on-site meals served in a common dining room, plus one or more of such services as on-site medical/nursing services, personal care, or housekeeping" (p. 239).

In contrast, assisted or "sheltered" housing as operated in many states offers a more extensive package of services with an emphasis on meals and personal care. Some states are instituting subsidized assisted housing in single-family homes. Assisted housing helps with personal needs, but is not a care facility. Individual residents remain responsible for their own care with support services available as needed. Assisted housing does not have ongoing health services.

The growth in congregate housing has come long after the availability of both independent-living housing situations and institutional settings. Congregate housing was authorized in 1970 in the congregate housing provision of the Housing and Urban Development Act. By 1990, almost $50 million had been appropriated for congregate services. These funds supported services for approximately 1,900 residents living in 60 projects. Although no funds for new congregate housing efforts have been made available since 1995, expiring grants have been continued on a year-to-year basis. Given the increasingly older population of the 202 units, it is not surprising that many of the projects are interested in providing either congregate meals or housekeeping services for residents.

The idea of locating extensive services in 202 housing is not new. Projects in some communities include a variety of services operated and financed by state or local agencies. Operating funds can now be used to hire service coordinators. In Section 202 projects with Congregate Housing Services Programs, the salary for the services coordinator must be taken from operating funds rather than the congregate service budget. The service coordinator provides referrals, support, and linkages for tenants with needs. HUD allows service coordinators in housing projects.

Despite the need for congregate services in many housing facilities, caution has been recommended in their development. As Lawton (1976) pointed out: "An environment that demands active behavior from its inhabitants facilitates maintenance of independent function. Conversely, the presence of too easily accessible services will erode independence among those who are still relatively competent" (p. 240).

Whatever the validity of this belief, providing additional services does require additional money that cannot be fully recouped from fees charged the residents. Further, the provision of these services could possibly duplicate other community resources.

Foster Care

For many years, the concept of foster care has been familiar to those who work with children, but the service has been made available to the elderly only since the early 1970s. In 1996, an estimated 60,000 state-licensed adult foster care facilities were in operation (Advisory Panel on Alzheimer's Disease, 1996). The number of these facilities continues to grow. In one Michigan county, St. Clair, 91 foster care homes were in operation during 2003. This high number represented one home for every 202 individuals in the county over the age of 65 (Chapin, 2003).

Foster care focuses on a population that cannot sustain full independence. It thus attempts to prolong independence and delay institutionalization. Foster care is a specialized form of sheltered housing whereby the client is placed in a new setting that has family supports. Although Newman and Sherman (1977) describe foster care as a system "for persons in need of care and protection in a substitute family setting for a planned period of time" (p. 436), a more recent survey of the literature has found at least six definitions of foster family care (Hudson, Dennis, Nutter, Galaway, & Richardson, 1994). These definitions differ in what they regard as a family and how many individuals fit into this family unit. It is fair to say, however, that in most foster care programs, the number of older persons per family unit is small, probably averaging not more than four. Louisiana defines adult foster care as "a private residence with the approved capacity to receive six or fewer adults who are aged, emotionally disturbed, developmentally disabled, or physically handicapped who require supervision on an ongoing basis but who do not require continuous nursing care" (State of Louisiana, 1997).

Foster care programs are generally administered by local departments of social services and have relied heavily on Title XX funds for operation. Strict income limitations were attached to the Title XX funding, which made moderate- or high-income elderly ineligible for foster care through Title XX funding. Although more limited, monies are also available through state departments of health or mental health and through the Veterans Administration. More liberal income policies are in effect when funds from these sources are being used. In some programs, the foster family is paid a percentage of the SSI check directly by the recipient of the foster care. In these cases, the foster family does not always break even on the costs. Eligible homes are usually solicited through appeals to the general public. After eligibility is determined, the foster family is paid a fee, plus certain expenses, for the care of the older person. One of the limitations to expanding this program is in the recruitment of families.

Foster care has been found to be especially effective for older discharged mental patients. The largest foster care program in the United States is run by the Veterans Administration. An important test of the utility of foster care for individuals who would otherwise be placed in nursing homes has been conducted in Massachusetts and in Maryland since 1978. In this program, individuals being discharged from the hospital are assigned randomly either to foster care homes or to nursing home care in order to assess the relative social and cost effectiveness of these two service modalities. Caretakers are paid $350–$500 per month. The cost of the Community Care program has been 32% below that of nursing-home care.

The participants in the program showed better or improved functioning on the Activities of Daily Living and better mental status scores than controls in nursing homes. The Community Care program participants also were more likely to achieve the nursing goals set for them. In contrast, nursing home residents were more involved in a variety of social activities and had higher life satisfaction scores at the end of 1 year (Oktay & Volland, 1987). A state-run foster care program in Massachusetts, Adult Family Care, matches older people with families in communities. As part of this effort, a Massachusetts Council for Adult Foster Care has been organized. As Oktay and Volland (1981) note, foster care cannot be used for all patients, some of whom are too hostile, demanding, or ill to be placed with a non-family caregiver. In some cases, patients or their families resist the idea of foster home care, either because it is new or the family feels that the care provided cannot be intensive enough to meet their relative's needs. Given the findings on social activities, it is also important to consider whether foster care results in social isolation of older persons in communities where social activities and transportation are not adequate.

Board and Care and Domiciliaries

Board and care homes are widely available, but there has been little information available about these facilities. Because there are no national regulations governing this level of care, each state has adopted its own terminology and regulations that govern the type of care given. Probably the best definition for this general level of care is contained in the Colorado regulations:

> An establishment operated and maintained to provide residential accommodation, personal services and social care to individuals who are not related to the licensee, and who, because of impaired capacity for self-care, elect or require protective living accommodations but who do not have an illness, injury, or disability for which regular medical care and 24-hour nursing services are required. [Glasscote et al., 1976, p. 58]

In summary, this level of care is primarily personal and custodial. Regulations for board and care homes usually require that

- local and fire safety codes be met;
- there be a full-time administrator responsible for the supervision of staff, residents, and safety;
- nursing personnel be on call most of the time; and
- there be facilities for occasional distribution of medication.

Board and care homes may be called "foster care," "residential care," "sheltered care," or even "assisted living." They usually have no more than 10 residents. These homes usually provide assistance to the older person with the activities of daily living, supervision of medications, laundry and linens, cleaning services, and protective supervision (Reisacher & Hornboster, 1995). As Reisacher and Hornboster make clear, board and care residences are neither nursing homes, congregate housing, nor shared housing or rooming houses. Although at least 30,000 licensed homes have been identified in studies (Hawes, Wildfire, & Lux, 1993; Lewin/ICF and James Bell Associates, 1990), there are estimates that an almost equal number of unlicensed homes exists (U.S. House of Representatives, Subcommittee on Health and Long-Term Care Policy, 1989). The licensed homes provide over 600,000 beds (Advisory Panel on Alzheimer's Disease, 1996). As Lyon (1997) notes, board and care homes predominantly serve low-income older persons who have major functional impairments and cannot rely on family resources to provide care.

Residents of board and care homes are usually required to arrange for their own medical care and, in many instances, provide for their own social activities. In effect, this level of care provides a protected environment, meals, and some personal care services, but does not restrict or organize the activities of the residents. Many low-income board-and-care residents are able to pay for care through their SSI checks. A 1991 study found that 90% of board and care homes were private and two-third were for-profit facilities. As expected, the majority (66%) of residents

were older women, two-thirds of whom were over the age of 65, and a
quarter of the residents were over the age of 85 (Assistant Secretary for
Planning and Evaluation, 1991).

Domiciliaries and homes for the aged are primarily nonprofit and often church-sponsored homes that provide personal care, but require that
persons entering be healthy. These homes go well beyond the standards
set by the various states in that they usually provide comprehensive activities, social services, and personal care programs. Many of the residents
have private rooms, and rarely are there more than two people in each
room. Residents can select activities that are offered and are free to come
and go as desired. These facilities can be small, often accommodating as
few as 50 residents, but in some cases are large enough to accommodate
as many as 300. Attached to many of these homes for the aged are intermediate care or skilled care nursing units to provide appropriate medical
treatment for those who need such care. Depending on the size of the facility, the home will either be able to continue to care for a resident who
needs medical care on a regular basis, or will transfer that person to a regular skilled or intermediate care facility.

Retirement Communities

One of the more recent phenomena developing as a result of the large
number of people who are retiring, particularly with good retirement incomes, is the retirement community. Retirement communities can range
from small mobile home subdivisions to sizable communities like Sun
City, Arizona. The communities can include apartments, semidetached
houses, and units that can be purchased or rented. Beyond the living units
themselves, varying forms of recreation and supportive services can be offered. The country's first development for senior citizens—Youngstown,
Arizona—was founded in 1954 and incorporated as a retirement community in 1960.

Most retirement communities have age as the key entrance requirement. Most communities that use the term "Active Retirement Living"
limit the ownership of homes to individuals over age 55. Other members
of the family must be at least 45 years of age and no residents can be under the age of 18. The general characteristics of retirement communities
include entrance requirements, complete community planning, and relatively low-cost housing, coupled with high levels of amenities. The concept
of low-cost housing, however, is not universal in retirement communities.

Retirement communities such as Sun City have extensive recreation
facilities. The usual construction pattern is of single-family attached and
detached houses in cul-de-sac arrangements, with the clubhouse as the
focal point.

One example of a successful retirement community is Leisure World in Laguna Hills, California. Begun in 1963, by spring 1977, it had nearly 12,000 residences and a population of 19,000. Leisure World was designed to provide security, quick accessibility to good health care, good nearby shopping, good transportation, excellent facilities for recreation and adult education and additional activities to ensure freedom from boredom (Leisure World, 1977).

The importance of security in a retirement community is illustrated in the efforts Leisure World has made:

> Hundreds of Leisure World residents say one of the principal reasons they came to live in Leisure World is security. . . . The entire residential area is surrounded by about 8.5 miles of six-foot wall or fence. In some places the wall is topped by barbed wire. Entrance to the residential areas is only through one of eleven guarded gates. Cars of residents have a special symbol attached to the front bumper; all others are stopped for identification and for permission by a resident to pass through . . . a security force of 255 officers is backed up by full-time, armed officers who have specific police training. [Leisure World, 1977, p. 9]

The facilities at Leisure World are extensive. Minibuses circulate over 11 routes, fare-free, carrying 88,000 passengers a month. There are five clubhouses, concerts, movies, stage presentations, and 167 clubs and organizations. The enormous sports and recreational opportunities range from swimming pools and horseback riding to a variety of crafts facilities. All of the activities offered by Leisure World are free to residents except golf and horseback riding. Health facilities are available but on a fee-for-service basis. The success of Leisure World in Laguna Beach is evidenced by the fact that the houses are sold by lottery drawn from the extensive waiting list.

Despite potentially large purchase costs and monthly maintenance fees, retirement communities are growing in popularity, particularly because they offer security, recreation, good housing, and social opportunities with neighbors of a similar age. Researchers commenting on a survey of residents in a number of retirement communities note:

> Most persons living in a retirement community have weighed the advantages and disadvantages of this life style. The evidence gathered on thirty-six communities suggests that there is a high amount of satisfaction with their choice. Despite problems or uncertainties about land ownership these communities deliver the kind of environment that their residents desire. [Streib, LaGreca, & Folts, 1986, pp. 101–102]

Although the pattern may change as the residents age, many retirement communities do not provide extensive services for their residents.

The CARES volunteer organization in Crestwood Village, New Jersey, provides transportation and free medical equipment to residents when needed.

"Continuing care retirement communities" or "life care communities" are more oriented to service provision for residents. Life care communities offer three types of contracts:

- An "extensive contract" provides unlimited nursing care.
- A moderate contract provides a specific amount of nursing care. After the limits of this amount of care are reached, additional care is provided for a fee.
- A charge is levied for all services (fee for service).

"Life care communities" include contracts that guarantee to provide all levels of care for the residents (Episcopal Homes Foundation, 2004).

These communities grew rapidly during the 1980s and guarantee to provide care for residents throughout the remaining years of their life, regardless of their physical condition. In many cases, residents pay a large entrance fee that may be as high as $200,000. In addition, there is a monthly charge of $1,000 to $2,500 based on the size of the apartment, its location, amenities provided in the community, and number of individuals living in the apartment (Health Insurance Information, 2002). As in many life care communities, these monthly charges do not cover most nursing home costs. Some life care communities guarantee to return a specific percentage of the entrance fee to the individual's estate, whereas others retain the whole fee.

Because of the long-term care nature of the services guaranteed, financial demands on life care communities are extensive. Some life care communities have failed because of inadequate financial resources, and some have had to raise the monthly resident charges drastically to meet their operating costs. In response, states have begun to scrutinize the economic resources of proposed life care developers, and 30 states now regulate these communities. Life care communities based purely on rental payments are also becoming available. In general, the resident population of life care communities tends to be over 75 years of age.

Recently, in order to broaden the market for these communities, there has been a movement away from entrance fees to communities that only charge monthly fees; these are adjusted according to the service needs of the residents. Under this plan individuals who require nursing care pay a higher monthly fee than other residents. As continuing care communities have grown in number, they have also begun to vary in what they offer. Whereas some provide nursing care on the premises, others are linked to nursing homes, or guarantee a resident priority in obtaining a nursing home bed (Lewin, 1990). As these communities are expected to grow in number, the development by hotel chains and nursing home firms clearly targets an affluent segment of the older population.

Although the discussion of retirement communities usually focuses on new planned developments, there has also been the movement toward what is labeled as "naturally occurring retirement communities." These communities come into existence as the residents of a community or housing complex grow older but stay in their own homes. The result is a large proportion of older persons in the area. In 1994, New York State began to provide supportive services for these types of retirement communities. The services are provided in housing developments built with government subsidies or loans but not specially built to serve older persons. In addition, older residents must occupy 50% of the units. In the 14 Naturally Occurring Retirement Communities, a variety of services, ranging from case management to health care, are provided for residents (Pine & Pine, 2002).

Shared and Accessory Housing

One seemingly simple approach to meeting the housing needs of older people is the "matching" of individuals who have similar housing needs. Although this may be a diverse group, including single younger individuals, this type of effort may enable older persons who require housing to find individuals with whom they can share homes. As housing costs continue to escalate and rental housing becomes scarcer, these types of matching efforts by local social services agencies have proliferated. A survey of 252 home sharing matches found a very positive feeling about home sharing among respondents. It reduced financial problems of the home sharers and promoted greater feelings of safety and less loneliness (Bergman, 1994). Shared housing can run into problems with zoning regulations that may restrict housing in an area to "families." Individuals living in shared housing are now eligible for the Section 8 program.

Existing Housing Certificate Program

Accessory housing utilizes parts of single-family homes as separate apartments for older relatives. "Granny flats," or Elder Cottage Housing Opportunities (ECHO) units, have been adopted from Australia. These freestanding manufactured homes are adjacent to existing single-family units, usually homes owned by children of the older individual living in the ECHO facility. Although ECHO units can be very cost effective, they also raise zoning issues in many residential communities zoned exclusively for single-family homes. ECHO housing units are now eligible for Section 202 financing.

Home Equity Programs

Many older people are "house rich and cash poor"; that is, they have a great deal of money invested in their homes. This is true of older persons at all income levels: 23% of elderly homeowners below the poverty line have over $50,000 equity in their homes (Fairbanks, 1990). Unfortunately, this money is not accessible unless the house is sold, a step that many older families do not want to take.

Many older people also find rising property taxes a difficult financial burden. Legislation that limits property taxes for older people can be vital in allowing homeowners to stay in their houses. One such program is a "circuit breaker" that prevents property taxes from rising above a percentage of the older person's income ("threshold programs"). Sliding scale programs rebate a percentage of property taxes to older persons, the percentage being determined by the older person's income. Thirty states have instituted some form of this tax relief. In addition, 17 states allow property taxes to be deferred until the death of the older person or the sale of his or her property.

Home equity conversion is a more ambitious effort to make available the equity older people have in their homes. Since 1980 a variety of programs, most commonly referred to as "reverse mortgages," have become available. By 1994, they were being used by 10,000 persons over the age of 62 (Bary, 1994). In 1995, Fannie Mae (formerly the Federal National Mortgage Association) began to offer reverse mortgages. Between 2003 and 2004, the number of reverse mortgages increased 112%. Along with their increased popularity, the financial problems of many seniors encouraged the use of this income source (*Senior Journal,* 2004). With a reverse mortgage, homeowners can stay in their own homes and use the funds they receive from a bank to cover other important expenses, including health care. The amount homeowners receive is based on the equity in their home and their age. A 75-year-old individual with a home valued at $100,000 can receive a monthly payment of $363 (Romano, 1996). The loan is paid back when the homeowner dies or moves through the sale of the house.

High interest rates and fees charged by some banks have raised questions about the value of these reverse mortgages for many older homeowners. These fees are substantially higher than those charged for conventional loans. The origination fee ("points") can range from 1–3% followed by closing costs of $1,700. In 1994, one lender in California was sued by homeowners incensed by its interest rates and fees (Bary, 1994). Individuals not planning to remain in their home for a long period after assuming a reverse mortgage can find this form of loan very expensive. In Maryland, a 75-year-old homeowner obtained a reverse mortgage that provided $568 per month. If the homeowner left this property after two years, he or she would have paid 50.22% in order to receive $13,000 (Lohse, 1995). There are also potential problems with reverse mortgages stemming from depreciation in home values that could make it difficult to recoup the loan from the sale of the home.

Fannie Mae began an innovation in the use of reverse mortgages in 1997. The "Our Home Keeper for Home" program allows individuals over the age of 62 to use reverse mortgages to buy a home. Fannie Mae regards this program as an opportunity for older individuals to relocate in order to be nearer family members or to live in another area of the country. Another innovative program is the co-housing village in Berkeley, California (Stock, 1997). In this model, residents manage their community and share dinners a few times a week. In contrast to age-restricted retirement communities, the small Berkeley community is age integrated. With no private lawns, the cottages and two-family townhouses ranged in price from $125,000 to $220,000. The variety of diverse housing programs available to older people can be expected to increase during the next decade.

REFERENCES

AARP. (2001). *A summary of federal rental housing programs.* Retrieved April 19, 2004, from http//research.aarp.org/il/fs85_housing.html

Abshier, G., Davis, Q., Jans, S., & Petranek, C. (1977). *Evaluation of the Cape-Smile home repair program.* Evansville, IN: Indiana State University.

Advisory Panel on Alzheimer's Disease. (1996). *Alzheimer's disease and related dementias: Report to Congress.* Washington, DC: U.S. Government Printing Office.

American Association of Retired Persons. (n.d.). *Understanding senior housing.* Washington, DC: Author.

Assistant Secretary for Planning and Evaluation. (1991). *ASPE research notes. Licensed board and care homes: Preliminary findings from the 1991 National Health Providers Study.* Retrieved September 26, 2004, from http://www.aspe.hhs.gov/daltcp/reports/rn06.htm

Bary, A. (1994, July 4). Reversals of fortune. *Barrons,* pp. 23–24.

Bergman, G. (1994). Shared housing: Not only for the rent. *Aging Today, 15,* 1, 4.

Chapin, B. (2003, October 11). More elderly choose foster homes. *Times Herald.* Retrieved January 16, 2005, from http://www.thetimesherald.com/news/stories/20031011/localnews/434505.html

Episcopal Homes Foundation. (2004). *Retirement with life care.* Retrieved from http://www.lifecare.org/continuing_care_retirement.html

Fairbanks, J. (1990). Home equity conversion programs: A housing option for the "house-rich, cash-poor" elderly. *Clearinghouse, 23,* 481–487.

$5.2 billion for low-income senior housing not reaching the elderly: Why?: Hearing before the Senate Special Committee, 108th Congress. (2003). Testimony of David Wood.

Glasscote, R., Biegel, A., Jr., Clark, E., Cox, B., Wiper, J. R., Gudeman, J. E., et al. (1976). *Old folks at homes.* Washington, DC: American Psychiatric Association and the Mental Health Association.

Government Accountability Office. (2005). *Elderly housing: Federal housing programs that offer assistance for the elderly.* Washington, DC: Author.

Hawes, C., Wildfire, J., & Lux, L. (1993). *National summary: The regulation of board and care homes: Results of a survey in the 50 states and the District of Columbia.* Washington, DC: American Association of Retired Persons.

Health Insurance Information. (2002). *Continuing care retirement communities or life care for long-term care.* Retrieved September 26, 2004, from http://www.healthinsurance.info/HICCR.HTM

Hudson, J., Dennis, D., Nutter, R., Galaway, G., & Richardson, B. (1994). Foster family care for elders. *Adult Residential Care Journal, 8,* 65–76.

Lawton, M. (1976). The relative impact of congregate and traditional housing on elderly tenants. *The Gerontologist, 16,* 237–242.

Leger, M., & Kennedy, S. (1990). *Final comprehensive report of the freestanding housing voucher demonstration: Vol. 1.* Washington, DC: U.S. Department of Housing and Urban Development.

Leisure World. (1977). Laguna Hills, CA: Leisure World.

Lewin, T. (1990, December 2). How needs, and market, for care have changed. *New York Times,* p. A36.

Lewin/ICF Inc. & James Bell Associates. (1990). *Descriptions of supplemental information on board and care homes included in the update of the National Health Provider Inventory.* Washington, DC: U.S. Department of Health and Human Services.

Lohse, D. (1995, November 24). Help for cash-poor, home-rich seniors at a price. *Wall Street Journal,* pp. C1, 15.

Lyon, S. (1997). Impact of regulation and financing on small board and care homes in Maryland. *Journal of Aging and Social Policy, 9,* 37–50.

McCleary, K. (1986). Minor repairs for older homeowners. *Aging, 352,* 2–5.

McIlwain, J. (2004). Cited in W. Smith, The good life in the big city. *AARP Bulletin, 45*(6), 4–8.

Mollica, R. (2003). Coordinating services across the continuum of health, housing and supportive services. *Journal of Aging and Health, 15,* 165–188.

NAMI. (2004). *Threat to Section 8 continues.* Retrieved January 12, 2005, from http://www.nami.org/Template.cfm?Section=whats_new43&template=/ContentManagement/ContentDisplay.cfm&ContentID=19058

Newman, S., & Sherman, S. (1977). A survey of caretakers in adult foster homes. *The Gerontologist, 17,* 431–437.

Oktay, J., & Volland, P. (1981). Community care programs for the elderly. *Health and Social Work, 6,* 31–47.

Oktay, J., & Volland, P. (1987). Foster home care for the frail elderly as an alternative to nursing home care: An experimental evaluation. *American Journal of Public Health, 77,* 1505–1510.

Pine, P., & Pine, V. (2002). Naturally Occurring Retirement Community-Supportive Service Program: An example of devolution. *Journal of Aging and Social Policy, 14,* 181–193.

Reisacher, S., & Hornboster, J. (1995). *A home away from home.* Washington, DC: American Association of Retired Persons.

Retsinas, J., & Retsinas, N. (1992). Housing loopholes may hurt elders. *Aging Today, 13,* 1,2.

Romano, J. (1996, June 23). For reverse mortgages, a Fannie Mae imprimatur. *New York Times,* p. A19.

Senior Journal. (2004). Reverse mortgages up 112% from year ago. Retrieved September 26, 2004, from http://wwww,seniorjournal.com.NEWS/ReverseMortgage/4-04-12Up.htm

State of Louisiana. (1997). *Chapter 24-A: The Adult Foster Care Facility Licensing Act.* Baton Rouge, LA: Author.

Stock, R. (1997, December 18). Living independently in old age, without going it alone. *New York Times,* p. B10.

Streib, G., LaGreca, A., & Folts, W. (1986). Retirement communities: People, planning, prospects. In R. Newcomer, M. Lawton, & T. Byerts (Eds.), *Housing an aging society* (pp. 94–103). New York: Van Nostrand Reinhold.

U.S. Department of Housing and Urban Development. (1973). *Housing in the seventies.* Washington, DC: U.S. Government Printing Office.

U.S. Department of Housing and Urban Development. (1999). *Recent research results: New plan addresses housing needs of elderly.* Retrieved May 3, 2004, from http://www.huduser.org/periodicals/rrr/rrr8_99/rrrr8_99art4.html

U.S. Department of Housing and Urban Development. (2000). *Recent research results: New facts about home housing assistance by housing programs.* Retrieved September 12, 2004, from http://www.huduser.org/perodicals/rrrr/rrr_10_2000/1000_6.html

U.S. Department of Housing and Urban Development. (2004a). *CDBG grantee reported accomplishments.* Retrieved January 16, 2005, from http://www.hud.gov/offices/cpd/communitydevelopment/library/accomplishments/index.cfm

U.S. Department of Housing and Urban Development. (2004b). *A picture of subsidized households: Summary of the United States.* Retrieved May 3, 2004, from http://www.huduser.org/datasets/assthsg/statedata98/HUD4US33.txt

U.S. General Accounting Office. (2003). *Report to the U.S. Senate Special Committee on Aging. Elderly housing: Project funding and other factors delay assistance to needy households.* Washington, DC: U.S. Government Printing Office.

U.S. House of Representatives, Select Committee on Aging. (1976). *Elderly housing overview: HUD's inaction.* Washington, DC: U.S. Government Printing Office.

U.S. House of Representatives, Subcommittee on Health and Long-Term Care Policy. (1989). *Board and care homes in America: A national tragedy.* Washington, DC: U.S. Government Printing Office.

U.S. Senate, Special Committee on Aging. (1975). *HUD's response to the housing needs of senior citizens.* Washington, DC: U.S. Government Printing Office.

U.S. Senate, Special Committee on Aging. (1990). *Developments in aging: 1989,* *Vol. 2.* Washington, DC: U.S. Government Printing Office.

U.S. Senate, Special Committee on Aging. (1991). *Developments in aging: 1990:* *Vol. 1.* Washington, DC: U.S. Government Printing Office.

Weichert, J. (n.d.). *Testimony to the U.S. Senate Committee on Banking, Housing and Urban Affairs.* Retrieved January 13, 2005, from http://www.hud.gov/offices/cir/100902w.cfm

CHAPTER THIRTEEN

In-Home Services

THE GROWTH OF IN-HOME SERVICES

Home care continues its development as a major program for the older American population and now accounts for 14% of Medicare expenditures (General Accounting Office, 1996). In recent years home care has represented one of the fastest growing components in Medicare expenditures.

Eligibility for home care depends on the individual's degree of disability, but defining disability is difficult because of the various measurement standards that are used. The number of Activities of Daily Living that individuals cannot perform without assistance is becoming more utilized as a disability standard. In 1999, the number of chronically disabled older adults was estimated at 7.1 million. Advances in medical technology and changes in life styles among older adults kept this number below what would have been expected if previous rates of chronic disability had been maintained, in which case an estimated 9.2 million older adults would have been classified as chronically disabled in 1999 (Manton and Gui, 2001).

In-home services are provided to individuals who live in their own homes or apartments. The hope is that these services can "through coordinated planning, evaluation and follow-up procedures, provide for medical, nursing, social and related services to selected persons . . . with a view toward shortening the length of hospital stay, speeding recovery, or preventing inappropriate institutionalization" (U.S. Senate, Special Committee on Aging, 1972, p. 25).

In-home services to the elderly are approximately evenly divided between health and welfare agencies, a phenomenon that has resulted from the parallel, but relatively independent, growth of social and health services to the homebound. Welfare agencies were the first to offer in-home services. In the early 1900s, private charitable family agencies provided homemakers to care for children whose mother was sick. During the 1930s, poor and unemployed women were hired as housekeepers for other poor persons who were in need of the service.

With the introduction of Medicare and Medicaid in the mid-1960s, the emphasis shifted from family and child care to serving the elderly. With this shift in recipient population came a shift in the type of care given, from home maintenance to personal care. The care of the sick, elderly person required an emphasis on personal care, and Medicare and Medicaid reimbursed only for the personal care aspects of in-home work.

The growth of agencies providing home health services has been remarkable. By 2003, there were 7,000 Medicaid-certified home health agencies. The overwhelming proportion (83%) of this growth has been among for-profit agencies (General Accounting Office, 1996). In addition to these agencies, an estimated 3,700 to 6,000 agencies were providing services, although not certified by Medicare. In 1996, almost 2 million home visits to older persons were recorded. Among these clients, 46% were between the ages of 75 and 84 and 25% over the age of 85 (National Center for Health Statistics, 2000).

The diversity of services and service providers makes it difficult to guarantee the quality of in-home services. The 1992 OAA amendments required State Units on Aging to monitor the quality of in-home services. In addition, the amendments add a section to Title III that guarantees the rights of clients of in-home services. These include the right to be informed in advance about a service, participate in its planning, voice grievances about its delivery, be treated with respect, have records treated as confidential, and be informed of rights under the OAA [Section 314].

Health agencies—long established to provide health services in community and institutional settings—started to add home health aid to their in-home services when reimbursements through Medicaid and Medicare became available. Skilled nursing care had been available through health agencies for some time before the new funding became accessible. With the new funding, welfare agencies offering homemaking and health agencies offering home health aid began offering the same or similar basic services. Both personal and homemaking services are required to enable persons to remain in their own homes. Because of the overlapping of personal and homemaking services by social and health agencies, a single person (homemaker or home health aide) can provide both services.

SERVICE PATTERNS

In-home services are of several levels or types, all of which should be flexible and readily changed as the client's needs change. Because they are administered in the home of the client, in-home services are an extension of the individual's functioning. Because they are personalized to individual situations, there is a potential need to change their components as persons respond to the services being given. Thus, coordination of services is an integral element of successful in-home services. A smoothly functioning network of services must be available to ensure that the individual receives exactly what is needed at the time it is needed. Strong links and easy accessibility among the services are essential to ensure cooperation for the benefit of the client. For example, Baltimore coordinates 10 in-home service agencies through a central intake system so that a client can be matched with the most appropriate services. As needs change, the central intake system can continue to reassign the appropriate services.

Available in-home services can be grouped into three general categories, based on the level of intensity of service (U.S. Senate, Special Committee on Aging, 1972).

Intensive or Skilled Services

These services are ordered by a physician and provided under the supervision of a nurse. Skilled care is given to clients with such problems as cardiac difficulties, bone fractures, open wounds, diabetes, and terminal illnesses involving catheters and tube feedings. The services may require physician visits, regular visits by a nurse, and frequent physical and occupational therapy treatments. In addition, less technical services may be provided such as nutritional services, deliveries of drugs and medical supplies, home health equipment, transportation, and other diagnostic and therapeutic services that can be safely provided in the client's home.

The intensive or skilled level usually involves a complex grouping of services. The full services might not be needed for long, but modified amounts would probably be part of client planning for an extended period of time. Coordination is particularly important for this level of in-home services because of the potential for change and probable number of different service components that could be needed.

Personal Care or Intermediate Services

Clients eligible for personal care services are medically stable but need assistance with certain activities of daily living, such as bathing, ambulation, prescribed exercises, and medications. These services can be given to persons who are convalescing from acute illnesses or to persons with temporary disabilities related to a chronic illness, or as part of a chronic illness. Personal or intermediate care services can be given independently or in conjunction with skilled care.

Homemaker-Chore or Basic Services

These services involve light housekeeping, preparation of food, laundry services, and other maintenance activities that help sustain the client at home. In those circumstances where the clients can care for themselves but do not have the capacity to care for their personal environment, these basic services help sustain the home situation for them. Basic or chore services can be given in conjunction with both intermediate and skilled services and usually are given on an ongoing basis.

The key in-home service worker, particularly for both personal and homemaker-chore areas of service, is the homemaker-home health aide. Homemaker-home health aide services comprise the personal and home-making services needed to enable persons who cannot perform basic tasks for themselves to remain in their own homes. The basic duties performed include

- cleaning
- planning meals
- shopping for food
- preparing meals
- doing laundry
- changing bed linens
- bathing
- giving bed baths
- helping the person move from the bed to a chair
- helping the person perform simple exercises
- assisting with medications
- teaching new skills
- providing emotional support.

The homemaker-home health aide can perform personal care services, homemaking services, or both, as the training usually involves skill development in both areas. Although the number of trained aides has increased, it remains difficult to find qualified home health aides. A possible effect of this shortage could be the hiring of minimally qualified individuals to provide these important services to older persons.

Heavy house cleaning and simple home maintenance, such as painting and simple carpentry repairs, are usually performed by a person specifically employed for the purpose, and are not included in the homemaker-home health aide functions. Special programs matching high school or college students with the chore needs of older persons have enabled this type of work to be done. Usually, the older person pays a minimum wage for the services, as they are not covered under most funding programs.

An attempt to develop intensive services for seriously disabled older individuals without relocating them outside their own homes is exemplified by the Nursing Home Without Walls programs in New York State. This program was begun in 1977 and designed to be an alternative to institutionalization (Cardillo, Horton, & Luther, 1988). Individuals accepted into the program are provided a wide range of services comparable to those offered in a nursing home. The services are available on a 24-hour, 7-day-a-week basis and are offered through hospitals, residential health care facilities, and certified home health agencies. An older person assessed as needing skilled nursing care is also evaluated to determine whether he or she has a suitable living environment at home for this program. If the environment is physically suitable, a plan is prepared. The costs of the program's services are capped at 75% of the average annual cost for nursing home care, although exceptions are made to this formula. In 2004, a local home health agency in western New York was serving 175 clients through this program (TLC Health Network, 2004).

SERVICE AGENCIES

In-home services are provided by a variety of agencies that are usually based in the community and defined by the source of the funding and the service specialty.

> An agency eligible to receive Medicare and Medicaid funds is a home health agency, a public or private agency which in addition to requirements for sound administration, adequate records, professional supervision, assessment and review, has as its primary function the provision of skilled nursing service and at least one additional therapeutic service. [U.S. Senate, Special Committee on Aging, 1972, p. 21].

The agency is thus defined by the type of service that it provides.

Home health agencies can be both hospital and community based, public, private nonprofit, or proprietary.

Home Care Units of Community Hospitals

These units have emerged as a part of the hospital program, primarily as a method of discharging patients as soon as appropriate. As a hospital affiliate, the patient can retain the same doctor and can move in and out of the hospital as needed for ongoing care. Hospital-based programs are particularly effective for terminally ill patients who can spend some time at home but who need a close affiliation with emergency health services. These home care units are staffed primarily by public health nurses and have on call the medical units from the hospital itself. These units provide primarily skilled-care services.

Departments of Social Services

Local departments of social services usually provide intermediate- and basic-level in-home services under their adult services units. Because their background is a welfare agency, these homemakers are more likely to be involved with household activities and to a lesser extent with personal care services.

Private Nonprofit Community Agencies

Included in this group are such agencies as Associated Catholic Charities, Jewish Family and Children's Services, Family and Children's Services, and Visiting Nursing Associations. These types of agencies provide home-maker-home health aides, nurses, and other in-home service workers as part of larger community-related programs. Each agency usually selects which specific service area it will provide, such as personal care services only or nursing services, and incorporates them into the other agency services being given.

Community Health Centers

Community health centers can provide some in-home services as part of their program. The in-home services are usually tied to those clients who are participating in the health center as an extension of services given.

Proprietary Agencies

Proprietary agencies, such as Upjohn, provide in-home services to the homebound on a fee-for-service basis. The services are usually at the skilled level of care and provided for short periods of time.

Funding

The most difficult problem in the delivery of in-home services is funding. Because of current funding restrictions, the demand for services far exceeds the supply. Further, the demand is primarily for those types of services that are not readily reimbursable through the available funding sources. The community and institutional agencies that provide the services are available and prepared to deliver the services if the repayment mechanism is available for reimbursement. The greatest unmet need for in-home services is for those with long-term disabilities and for the chronically ill whose conditions are not likely to improve quickly.

There are five basic ways for payment of in-home services. The first—client fees—is used by most agencies that provide in-home services. Voluntary agencies are more likely to offer sliding-scale fee schedules because they are usually supported in part through contributions from individuals, religious groups, community groups, disease-related groups, or United Way fundraising organizations.

The second payment method—Medicare—is used by agencies that provide health-related services in situations where the client and the service meet Medicare eligibility requirements. In order to be eligible for Medicare reimbursement, the service must be given by a home health agency which has, as its primary function, the provision of skilled nursing service and at least one additional therapeutic service. The services that are reimbursable focus upon acute or short-term illnesses, not on chronic or custodial ones.

In addition, there are varying interpretations as to what is appropriate for reimbursement, interpretations that might be applied after the service has been given. Because of the potential unpredictability of Medicare reimbursements, agencies are often reluctant to give Medicare-reimbursed services other than those specifically defined as eligible. This makes it difficult for clients to receive appropriate services for their situations. Actual services provided under Medicare are restricted to home-bound patients (individuals unable to leave their home without the assistance of a person or a device such as a wheelchair or cane). Home care must be prescribed by the physician caring for the patient and the patient must require either intermittent skilled nursing care, physical therapy, or speech therapy (Leader, 1991). "Intermittent" care is defined as care provided at least once every 60 days, but once a patient meets Medicare eligibility, the services can be provided as long as they are medically necessary. As already noted, Medicare expenditures for home care continued to grow throughout the 1980s despite these restrictions.

Reimbursable services under Medicare include part-time or intermittent nursing care (under the supervision of a registered nurse); physical, occupational, and speech therapy; medical supplies; home health aide services; and counseling for social or emotional problems. The important services missing from this list are crucial personal and home maintenance services. Medicare-covered services have a maximum of 8 hours per day and 28 hours per week. A registered nurse for $20 to $60 per hour or a home aide for $7 to $15 per hour can mean an expense of $1,500 per week for a family attempting to maintain an impaired older person in the community (Alger, 1997).

Medicaid is the third payment method and is used by agencies that provide health-related services in situations where the client and the service meet Medicaid eligibility requirements. Unlike Medicare, in which every person age 65 and over is potentially eligible for the benefits, Medicaid is available only to those who meet strict income requirements. Although the actual income limit is determined within each state because Medicaid is partially financed by the states, the usual income limit is set to coincide with the SSI limit, plus whatever state aid for income is being given.

Home health care became a required service under Medicaid in 1970 and could be provided by the same agencies that are eligible for Medicare. Although the services provided under Medicaid vary among the states, Medicaid essentially covers nursing services, home health aide services, and medical supplies and equipment. Medicaid benefits do not require that skilled nursing care or therapy be given. Potentially eligible persons do not need prior hospitalization, nor is there a limit on the number of visits. Medicaid also allows personal care and non-medical services related to activities of daily living to be reimbursed. Section 1115 Medicaid-Waiver authority is being used by many states to fund in-home services for older persons. Despite this effort, at the end of the 1990s, more than 63% of Medicaid expenditures were being used for hospital or nursing home care (Palley, 2003). It is thus clear that Medicare is more likely to pay for in-home services whereas Medicaid is used primarily for institutional care. This is evident in the fact that 85% of all home health care for older persons in 2001 was paid for through Medicare funds (Federa Interagency Forum on Aging Related Statistics, 2004).

The Social Services Block Grant is also a source of funds for in-home services from public and private agencies. As already noted, these grant funds are allocated to the state departments of social services on the basis of population. Unlike Medicare and Medicaid, the services are not reviewed on a service-by-service basis for reimbursement. Home-based services, such as homemaker, home health aide, home management, personal care, consumer education, and financial counseling, were eligible services under the block grant. These services can be ongoing and are not restricted to a limited amount per year. However, the program is limited by the income eligibility of the client and the amount of money available to the public and private agencies for personnel to provide the services. Despite the opportunities for funding of in-home services under the block grant, only limited amounts of funds have been addressed to the needs of older clients and home health. In 2000, 6% of total Social Services Block grant funds were allocated to services for older persons living in the community (Administration for Children, Youth and Families, 2004).

The fifth payment source is Title III of the OAA, which provides monies for in-home services through the local Area Agencies on Aging.

The funds are made available to provide services designed to assist older individuals in avoiding institutionalization, including pre-institution evaluation and screening and home health services, homemaker services, shopping services, escort services, reader services, letter-writing services, and other similar services designed to assist such individuals to continue living independently in a home environment.

The funds can provide for a variety of services by both public and private agencies for both the chronically and acutely ill. The only eligibility requirement is that the recipient be 60 or over. Although there is no income restriction on the services, efforts are made to make most of them available to low-income elderly. The service limitation under Title III programs lies in the financial limits of the allocations themselves. Because eligible services are broadly defined under this act, efforts have been concentrated on using these funds and services for those people who are ineligible for them under the other funding programs.

RELATED SERVICES

There has been a growth in the number and types of formal support systems for the homebound that complement in-home services, or even substitute for these services when regular contact and visiting are all that are needed. Two such programs, reassurance and friendly visiting, are most frequently available, primarily as adjunct programs within senior centers or agencies providing other programs and services to the elderly. Gatekeeper initiatives are unobtrusive but valuable mechanisms for monitoring the well-being of community-based elderly.

Reassurance and Gatekeeper Services

As the number of elderly maintaining independent residence in the community continues to increase, a method for ensuring their daily well-being becomes vital. In housing specifically designed for seniors, systems that require turning off a hall light outside the apartment each morning can be used to indicate that the resident has not suffered any mishap during the previous day.

For individuals living in other types of residences, telephone reassurance has been stressed as a means of maintaining daily contact with older individuals. The telephone reassurance systems can be traced to the efforts of Grace McClure during the 1960s. After attempting to contact an elderly friend for 8 successive days, Mrs. McClure made a personal check of the friend's apartment and found her on the floor after having suffered a stroke. Mrs. McClure's subsequent efforts in Michigan resulted in a telephone reassurance service and replication of this type of service in many parts of the country (Conait, 1969).

In Pierce County, Washington, the telephone reassurance program uses trained volunteers who are responsible for calling the older persons once a day, 5 days a week. The calls are made at the same time each day. If no one answers the phone, checks are made with family and friends and eventually, if necessary, 911 is alerted (Senior Information and Assistance, Pierce County, 2004). The TRIAD program discussed in Chapter 8 has become a coordinator of telephone reassurance programs around the country. One possible and positive side effect of these services is the friendships that can form between volunteer callers and clients. This potential for friendships is being built into some services that utilize a buddy system. This approach depends on a team of approximately 10 people who utilize a daily round robin of calling. If the chain is broken on any day, the individual unable to make contact with the next person reports the problem to a central office, and a personal visit is made to the home.

If these services are well run, they are important links for the aging. More affluent elderly are now able to enroll in a service that enables them to hook their home into a central office. Failure to punch a code on a specially designed machine will result in a checkup visit to the home. Under these systems, central offices can be alerted to emergencies by either push-button codes or, in some cases, voice activation of the system. Social service agencies as well as hospitals are now making these automated systems available under a variety of fee schedules. The key link in the machine-based or telephone-based reassurance service is the reliability of the staff responsible for checking on the elderly client who fails to utilize the designated code or answer the phone. Because of this problem, few services are relying totally on relatives because of their possible unavailability at crucial times.

"Gatekeepers" are individuals who have frequent contact with older persons and can alert agencies about serious problems. In many rural areas, mail carriers are asked to alert a special office if they notice mail accumulating in an older person's mailbox. A customer representative for the utility company in Spokane, Washington, alerted Spokane Elder Services that a client had stopped paying her bills and appeared to be living in unsafe conditions. Other gatekeepers can include mail carriers, meter readers, bank tellers, clerks in stores, or pharmacists (Barnhill, 1997).

Visiting Services

Although they are now available in greater numbers, friendly visiting services have been operating in many cities for a long period of time. The visiting service in Chicago was begun in 1947. Friendly visitor services utilize volunteers to visit elderly individuals who are homebound. Visitors may chat with the older persons, read to them, help them with correspondence, or play chess and board games. Volunteers are trained to respond to the needs of the persons they visit, and they are matched with older persons according to shared interests and backgrounds. Partly as a result of these matching efforts, volunteers and the people they visit often become close friends (Cunneen-Lion, 1995).

Although they are most often oriented to community-based elderly, a friendly visitor service was begun in Maryland in 1977 to provide companionship for nursing home residents who did not receive regular visits by family and friends. One friendly visiting service utilized members of a senior citizens club as visitors. Programs around the country rely on volunteers of all ages to reach elderly who might otherwise be isolated from social contacts. In Los Altos, California, "cheergivers" visit selected residents of nursing homes weekly for an hour at a time (Cunneen-Lion, 1995).

Expansion of effective in-home services still hinges on the institution of funding mechanisms to make these services more reimbursable. Under the 1987 Older Americans Act amendments, a program of grants to individual states was authorized. The services that can be provided to frail elderly under this program are extensive. They include homemaker and home health aides as well as non-health services such as chore services, telephone reassurance, respite care in the home for family caretakers, and minimal physical modification of the home. Over half of these clients are from low-income backgrounds. Even with their expansion, it is questionable whether in-home services from formal providers can substitute for emotional support from family and friends.

REFERENCES

Administration for Children, Youth and Families. (2004). *Social Services Block Grant, 2000*. Retrieved October 21, 2004, from http://www.acf.hhs.gov/programs/ocs/ssbg/docs/ch300.htm

Alger, A. (1997, March 24). Nursing home or home nursing? *Forbes*, p. 160.

Barnhill, W. (1997). I was just passing by. *AARP Bulletin, 38*, 2, 10.

Cardillo, A., Horton, R., & Luther, C. (1988). *Nursing Home Without Walls Program: A decade of quality care at home for NY's aged and disabled*. Albany: New York State Senate Health Committee.

Conait, M. (1969). *Guidelines for telephone reassurance services*. Ann Arbor, MI: Univ. of Michigan, Institute of Gerontology.

Cunneen-Lion, M. (1995, July 31). Friendly visitors bring kindness, friendship to Los Altos seniors. *Los Altos Town Crier*. Retrieved October 21, 2004, from http://latc.com/1995/07/31/community/community4.html

Federal Interagency Forum on Aging Related Statistics. (2004). *Sources of payment for health care services*. Retrieved December 21, 2004, from http://www.agingstats.gov/chartbook2004/healthcare.html#Indicator%2033

General Accounting Office. (1996). *Medicare: Home health utilization expands while program controls deteriorate.* Washington, DC: Author.

Leader, S. (1991). *Medicare's home health benefit: Eligibility, utilization, and expenditures.* Washington, DC: Public Policy Institute, American Association of Retired Persons.

Manton, K., & Gui, X. (2001). *Changes in the prevalence of chronic disability in the United States Black and nonblack population above age 65 from 1982 to 1999.* Chapel Hill, NC: Duke University Center for Demographic Studies. Retrieved October 7, 2004, from http://www.advamed.org/VOT/value/advamed3.pdf

National Center for Health Statistics. (2000). *Characteristics of elderly home health care users: Data from the 1996 National Home and Hospice Care Survey.* Advance Data, No. 309.

Palley, H. (2003). Long-term care policy for older Americans: Building a continuum of care. *Journal of Health and Social Policy, 16*(3), 7–18.

Senior Information and Assistance, Pierce County. (2004). *Telephone reassurance program.* Retrieved on October 18, 2004, from http://www.co.pierce.wa.us

TLC Health Network. (2004). *What's new at TLC Health: Home health care offers alternative to nursing homes.* Retrieved October 21, 2004, from http://www.wnynetworks.com/tlchealth/whatsnew.php3

U.S. Senate, Special Committee on Aging. (1972). *Home health services in the United States.* Washington, DC: U.S. Government Printing Office.

CHAPTER FOURTEEN

Adult Day Care

THE ROOTS OF DAY CARE

Dependency and Aging

It is unfortunate that day care services for the elderly often seem to resemble services for children. Although the two programs may be similar in some aspects, services for the aged should not be based on viewing the elderly as childlike. As one advocate for adult day care urged in the early years of this service's development:

> We object to the comparison to child care because it is inaccurate. We are not a place where people are left in safety as children are left, until someone is ready to "pick them up" again. Our services have an objective, and those who are consumers are not children. They are adults who may be limited for shorter or longer periods of time in their capacities for total self-care—but they are participants in their own care programs with everything that the term implies. [Lupu, cited in Trager, 1976, p. 6]

The common thread running through services for children and the elderly is dependency. Lupu (1976) argued, however, that dependency among the elderly and children stems from different sources. The elderly do not lack knowledge of "right and wrong" and have attained the skills necessary to conduct their everyday life. Dependency in the elderly usually stems from physical and mental impairments that make it difficult for them to continue to accomplish routine tasks successfully. These tasks may include activities of daily living (ADLs) such as dressing, bathing, using the bathroom, cooking, and self-feeding. The task of the day care center is to assist the individual in functioning as independently as possible given their physical and mental status.

A National Council on the Aging (NCOA) study defines day care as a

> community based group program designed to meet the needs of func-
> tionally impaired adults through an individual plan of care. It is a struc-
> tured, comprehensive program that provides a variety of health, social,
> and related support services in a protective setting during any part of a
> day but less than 24 hour care. [Behrens, 1986, p. 5]

A slightly different emphasis can be seen in the definition that emphasizes that

> adult day care centers provide a break (respite) to the caregiver while
> providing health services, therapeutic services and social activities for
> people with Alzheimer's disease and related dementia, chronic illnesses,
> traumatic brain injuries, developmental disabilities and other problems
> that increase their care needs. [ARCA National Respite Network and
> Resource Center, 2004]

History of Day Care

Day care is one possible response to the need for families to have a daily
respite from caring for an impaired older person. Kaplan (1976, pp.
7–10) summarized the basic assumptions about day care as a belief in (1)
"the intrinsic worth of living within one's community;" (2) the merit in
keeping the family together; (3) the beneficial nature of allowing a person
to continue independent living; and (4) independent living as beneficial in
the broader concept of social well-being for older persons and their families.

Day care for adults originated in Britain during the 1940s, when outpatient hospital centers for psychiatric patients were set up. These centers, located in psychiatric hospitals, were designed to decrease the
numbers of individuals who would require admittance to inpatient units.
By the late 1950s, the British had extended day care programs to include
geriatric patients; by 1969, 90 programs were already in operation.

In 1947, the first geriatric day hospital in the United States opened
under the auspices of the Menninger Clinic, and in 1949, a similar operation was begun at Yale (McCuan, 1973). Bolstered by the increased interest and funding for aging programs in the 1970s, day care programs
have expanded dramatically. In 1970, 15 day care centers were in existence. By 1999, more than 4,000 were operating (ARCA National
Respite Network and Resource Center, 2004). Even with this dramatic
increase, a federal report estimates that more than 10,000 centers are
needed to meet the needs of American elderly (Advisory Panel on
Alzheimer's Disease, 1996).

DAY CARE CLIENTS

Eligibility

Because of this short history, a variety of programs with varied focuses now fall under the day care rubric. Federal guidelines have not yet been set up to determine eligibility for federally funded day care programs. In 1974, Congress authorized demonstration day care programs. In its guidelines for these programs, the federal government defined day care as a program "provided under health leadership in an ambulatory care setting for adults who do not require 24-hour institutional care and yet, due to physical and/or mental impairment, are not capable of full-time independent living" (U.S. Health Resources Administration, 1974, p. 1).

An individual with physical and mental impairment was further defined under these guidelines as a "chronically ill or disabled adult whose illness or disability does not require 24-hour inpatient care but which in the absence of day-care service may precipitate admission to or prolonged stay in a hospital, nursing home or other long-term facility" (U.S. Health Resources Administration, 1974, p. 1). It is obvious that the major projected day care population is an at-risk group whose involvement in day care programs may provide enough support to enable them to remain out of long-term care institutions. Among existing programs, day care is not often used for individuals discharged from nursing homes.

Present Users

An Ohio study compared day care users and impaired elderly. Day care participants were more likely to be unmarried, living with other individuals, and in a physically more dependent position than impaired community elderly not involved with the day care program (Barresi & McConnell, 1984). Those who become caretakers as the elderly individual's physical or mental condition deteriorates may be the first to perceive the need for day care. Referrals to day care centers may come either from the families of elderly persons or from agencies or service providers who come into contact with the families and are aware of the centers. In contrast, the literature on nursing homes indicates that the majority of long-term residents have previously lived alone. It is therefore possible that day care clients differ from nursing home residents in the degree to which family members provide economic, social, and psychological support.

Adult day care clients can also be compared to individuals who use home health services. In a study of 62 adult day care users and 91 home health care users, the adult day care clients were found to be younger, have more problems with cognition, and need more supervision and assistance with activities of daily living (Dabelko and Balaswaym, 2000).

Individuals who come into day care programs from nursing homes are not in need of the 24-hour nursing services offered by these homes. The day care centers are expected to provide a range of services necessary to maintain the participants near their present level of functioning.

Evaluating Benefit to Clients

The ambiguities that now exist in definitions of day care create an initial difficulty in evaluating the effectiveness of these programs. If day care centers are maintenance oriented, it still may be difficult to evaluate the centers that enroll large numbers of seriously impaired individuals. Despite the extensive care a center may provide, deterioration, admission to nursing homes, or death is possible among these individuals. A broken hip, myocardial infarction, or organic brain syndrome may occur at any point in the impaired elderly person's day, occurrences that may be unaffected by attendance at a day care center. Although it is possible that the day care services may delay the onset of these conditions or deterioration in existing conditions, the use of adult day care has not been shown to have an effect on the health or mental health outcomes of clients (Weissert, Elston, Musliner, & Mutran, 1991). Adult day care centers have also not been found to delay nursing home placement (Zarit, Stephens, Townsend and Greene, 1998).

Eligibility for day care services as well as evaluation of the center's ability to meet its stated goals will be determined to a great extent by the range of services offered by the individual center. Thus the clients served and the criteria used for evaluation will differ among centers that are rehabilitation oriented and have multiple medical services, maintenance-oriented centers with many different services (not all offered on site), and centers that are socially oriented and have a minimum of medical services.

DAY CARE CENTER SERVICES

Program Outlines

The range of services that day care centers currently provide to maintain impaired clients at their optimal level of functioning is clear: screening for physical conditions; medical care (usually by arrangement with an outside physician); nursing care; occupational, physical, and recreational therapy; social work; transportation; meals; personal care (e.g., assistance in going to the toilet); educational programs; crafts; and counseling. In contrast to senior centers, day care services are not available on a drop-in basis. Clients are scheduled, usually on a minimal 2-day-per-week basis, but often on a full 5-day basis. Whereas many clients are ambulatory, day care centers endeavor to provide transportation and appropriately designed space to serve individuals confined to wheelchairs.

Most day care centers are small, typically serving 15–25 clients a day. This size helps to prevent the development of an institutional atmosphere. Centers are located in settings ranging from schools, apartments, and churches to hospitals and nursing homes. A random sample of adult day care in five states (Brasher, Estes, & Stuart, 1995) found that 45% of the centers were freestanding.

Clients usually arrive at the center between 9 and 10 A.M. and may have coffee before becoming involved in an individual or group project. A period of exercise matching the client's capability may be held before lunch, followed by a rest period and another group or individual project. These projects range from crafts and reading to dances and discussions. At any point in the day, appropriate counseling, nursing care, and medical-social services may be provided. Activities are conducted in accordance with the individual plan of care developed for each client upon his or her acceptance into the program. Clients are transported back to their residence in the late afternoon (3–4 p.m.). This schedule would not apply to centers that run an extended-hours program in the morning and afternoon. As would be expected, the staff–client ratio necessary to provide the individualized attention described here is high, averaging around 1:5 or 1:7 at most centers. In order to maintain the client's relationship with the community, many centers make extensive use of volunteers and emphasize frequent outings, including picnics, shopping, and trips.

Program and Client Emphasis

The major disagreement among day care advocates has revolved around the relative emphasis on particular services. This lack of consensus can be seen in the ambiguous guidelines for the 1974 demonstration programs:

> The essential elements of day care programs are directed towards meeting the health maintenance and restorative needs of participants. However, there are socialization elements which by overcoming the isolation often associated with illness in the aged and disabled are considered vital for the purpose of fostering and maintaining the maximum possible state of health and well being. [U.S. Health Resources Administration, 1974]

The relegation of socialization programs to the second sentence of these guidelines reflects uncertainty as to the importance of these elements in the day care program.

Unless federal or state guidelines clearly specify the outlines of day care services, the components emphasized will partially depend on the affiliation or sponsorships of the centers. Day care centers sponsored by Area Agencies on Aging may have a greater degree of emphasis on social rather than health components, depending for their health services on linkages with medical and nursing schools. Programs such as the Mosholu-Montefiore program in New York place a heavy emphasis on health components because of their strong relationship to major hospital facilities and, in the case of this particular program, because it uses space provided by the hospital. The actual ratio of health to social services depends on the requirements of funding sources. Trager (1976) succinctly summed up the problems that may result from viewing social and health components as distinct and separate day care entities:

> The development of centers which set policies and objectives in the context of treatment and physical restoration may tend to exclude those in need of some, but not all of these services. For those who are considered candidates for supervision and socialization, there may be a tendency to ignore essential health related services. Facilities which are treatment oriented may also tend to take on institutional characteristics and to make a "patient" of the participant—an aspect of institutional care which often is counterproductive in terms of the objectives of treatment. On the other hand, major emphasis on a supervision-socialization policy excludes consideration of restoration and rehabilitation possibilities which may appear to be relatively limited but are of great importance to the participant and such facilities might take on the characteristics of current institutions which are "holding facilities" and ignore essential health needs. [p. 16]

Adult day care centers can now be classified into three basic types:

- Adult day social care centers that provide activities, meals, and recreation. In these centers some health-related services may be provided.
- Adult day health care. These centers provide a greater range of health and therapeutic services. Many of their programs are directed to meeting the needs of older people with severe medical problems who may be at risk of placement in a nursing home
- Adult day care centers that specialize in providing health and social services for older persons with Alzheimer's disease or related problems.

In order to bring some coherence to adult day care, the National Adult Day Services Association has developed a set of "Standards and Guidelines," which includes specifications about varied levels of care that can be offered by day care centers.

RESPITE SERVICES

Closely related to day care, respite services are strongly advocated, but receive only limited financial support. Although there are questions as to whether the target of respite is a caregiver or care receiver, respite services usually offer relief to individuals who provide intensive day care for older relatives or even unrelated individuals. Respite care, it is hoped, can also delay the placement of the older person in a long-term care institution such as a nursing home. Respite care can be provided on a brief scheduled basis such as 3 hours per week or sporadically in an institutional setting (Family Caregiver Alliance, 2001). At the Pennsylvania Medical Center in Philadelphia, the "HotelHospital" program provides 8–12 beds in a 12-bed unit for temporary residents (Hegeman, 1993). In Rochester, New York, St. John's Home provides two private skilled nursing facility rooms for respite stays of 1 to 6 weeks (Hegeman). In New Jersey, respite care is provided for 2,800 clients over the age of 18 (Family Caregiver Alliance). Rather than having respite services provided through different state agencies that target varied populations, states such as Oregon and Wisconsin have adopted a "Lifespan" approach. Through the Lifespan effort, any clients with special needs are provided respite care through one agency charged with providing it to all state residents who need this service (Family Caregiver Alliance).

FUNDING

As the discussion of funding sources in Chapter 2 indicates, services for the aging are now being kept afloat through monies obtained from a number of sources. This is exemplified by day care, where a variety of federal, local, and private funds are used. At the federal level, Medicaid plays a dominant role in funding adult day care centers, but many centers also rely on fees paid by participants or their families.

In 1976, the Medical Services Administration issued guidelines designed to assist states in preparing regulations for reimbursable day care centers. Although the target population of these centers might not differ from the centers already described, the medical service requirements might be more extensive. Programs conducted by a hospital or those that are recognized as "clinics under state laws" are eligible for Medicaid reimbursements. Under the guidelines, the reimbursable medical services that day care centers might offer include:

1. Medical services supervised by a physician
2. Nursing services rendered by a professional nursing staff

3. Diagnostic services in addition to initial screening
4. Rehabilitation services including physical therapy, speech therapy, occupational therapy, and inhalation therapy
5. Pharmaceutical services
6. Podiatric services
7. Optometric services
8. Self-care services oriented toward the activities of daily living
9. Dental services
10. Social work services
11. Recreation therapy
12. Dietary services
13. Transportation services

Although existing centers may provide many of these services, provision of all of them is probably beyond the resources of many. The guidelines specify that the package of services available for any individual must be a combination of some or all of the elements listed. All of these services might be available in a center, but it is expected that the most complex medical services would be found in day hospital settings, because of the close hospital-staff linkages. In all centers, the guidelines stress screening of clients by a multidisciplinary team and the development of an individualized treatment plan.

Based on the guidelines, each state has the responsibility to establish and approve a required package of services for reimbursable day care and day hospital programs. Intense discussions have developed about the degree of medical support that will be required by the state to qualify a center for reimbursement.

Under the Social Services Block Grant, many day care centers were funded without the extensive medical services that may be required under Medicaid. Unfortunately, Social Services Block Grant funds are limited and based on annual population figures for each state. Social Service Block Grants are also allocated on the basis of public hearings, and plans are developed on a statewide level. Some states have not included day services for the elderly in their plans, whereas others have viewed block grant support only as seed money for programs. Programs that were instituted on the basis of the block grant allocation have now found that block grant funds are not always available to meet increasing inflationary costs. Some states have cut back individual program funding in order to distribute small amounts of money to a larger number of centers. In this way, the states hope to encourage a larger number of centers, but individual centers then have to scramble to meet the deficit imposed by the cuts in their funding.

COST-EFFECTIVENESS AND BENEFITS

Even before their social and psychological benefits have been determined, day care centers have had to face the question of their costliness. Unfortunately, cost-effectiveness studies fail to provide enough clarity to allow for a final determination of the financial question. Because of variations in services, costs may differ widely among centers. In Connecticut, the Connecticut Home Care Program for Elders pays centers $55 per day for each client in a medically oriented full-day adult day care program and $52 for a socially oriented program. The actual costs of the daily programs were estimated to average $72 (Niesz, 2004). In California, adult day care services offered through Loma Linda University charge $45 per day (Loma Linda Medical Center, 2003). A recreational adult day care program in Bellingham, Washington, charges $15 per day (Eastwood, 2004). Differences in services probably account for the wide variations in these costs.

A variety of questions can be asked about day care services:

1. Do day care centers enable impaired elderly to maintain residence in the community?
2. Do day care services improve or maintain their participants' level of physical or emotional functioning?
3. Do the centers increase the participants' independence in basic activities of daily living?
4. Do day care services prevent or postpone institutionalization of participants?
5. Do day care services improve or maintain the participants' interpersonal relationships with family and friends?
6. Do day care services assist individual participants in reestablishing their desired lifestyles or increasing their life satisfaction?
7. Do day care services offer support for family members involved in the care of an elderly individual?

Not all of the goals of adult day care centers are easily met. In part, this may be because older individuals and their caregivers wait too long before utilizing the centers. By the time individuals are involved with the center they are often too frail to benefit from many of its programs.

Whatever the limits of their effects on older participants, adult day care centers can have positive effects on their primary caregivers. Caregivers of individuals who used adult day care centers have been found to have lower scores on measures of stress and lesser degrees of depression or anger. These effects were found by the researchers to still be present one year after the initial study (Zarit et al., 1998).

Day care has established itself as an important component of the continuum of services for the aged. With day care programs available, the caregiver of an older person in the community has some alternatives to the often seemingly overwhelming burdens of care. The most appropriate model for day care programs will probably remain an issue related to the availability of other services in the community, such as home care, and the characteristics of the older population for whom the day care center is targeted. One consequence of an increased emphasis on health care services in adult day care centers would be higher program costs (Weisser et al., 1991). This could create difficulties for smaller centers and possibly result in some centers being unable to meet state regulations.

REFERENCES

Advisory Panel on Alzheimer's Disease. (1996). *Alzheimer's disease and related dementias: Report to Congress.* Washington, DC: U.S. Government Printing Office.

ARCA National Respite Network and Resource Center. (2004). *Factsheet Number 54. Adult day care: One form of respite for older adults.* Retrieved October 22, 2004, from http://www.archrespite.org/archfs54.htm

Barresi, C., & McConnell, D. (1984, November). *Discriminators of adult day care participation among retired elderly.* Paper presented at the Gerontological Society of America Annual Meeting, San Antonio, TX.

Behrens, R. (1986). *Adult day care in America.* Washington, DC: National Council on the Aging.

Brasher, J., Estes, C., & Stuart, M. (1995). Adult day care: A fragmented system of policy and funding streams. *Journal of Aging and Social Policy, 7,* 17–38.

Dabelko, H., & Balaswaym, S. (2000). Use of adult day services and home health services. *Home Health Care Quarterly, 18*(3), 65–79.

Eastwood, B. (2004, October 17). Day care can be for seniors too. *Daily News Tribune.* Retrieved October 27, 2004, from http://www.dailynewstribune.com/localRegional/view.bg?articleid=42893

Family Caregiver Alliance. (2001). *Respite care: State policy trends and model programs.* Retrieved October 29, 2004, from http://www.caregiver.org/caregiver/jsp/content/pdfs/op_2001_10_policybref_4.pdf

Hegeman, C. (1993). Models of institutional and community-based respite care. In L. Tepper & J. Toner (Eds.), *Respite care* (pp. 3–29). Philadelphia: Charles. Press.

Kaplan, J. (1976). Goals of day care. In E. Pfeiffer (Ed.), *Day care for older adults* (pp. 7–10). Durham, NC: Duke University Center for the Study of Aging and Human Development.

Loma Linda Medical Center. (2003). *Adult day services.* Retrieved October 27, 2004, from http://www.llu.edu/llumc/progserv/adultday/html

McCuan, E. R. (1973). *An evaluation of a geriatric day care center as a parallel service to institutional care.* Baltimore, MD: Levindale Geriatric Research Center.

Niesz, H. (2004). *OLR research program: Connecticut adult day care centers.* Retrieved October 27, 2004, from http://www.cga.state.ct.u/2004/rpt/2004-R-0774.htm

Trager, B. (1976). *Adult day facilities for treatment, health care and related services.* Washington, DC: U.S. Government Printing Office.

U.S. Health Resources Administration, Division of Long-Term Care. (1974). *Guidelines and definitions for day care centers under PL. 92-603.* Washington, DC: U.S. Government Printing Office.

Weissert, W., Elston, J., Musliner, C., & Mutran, E. (1991). Adult day care regulation: Deja vu all over again? *Journal of Health Politics, Policies, and Law, 16,* 51–67.

Zarit, S., Stephens, M., Townsend, M. A., & Greene, R. (1998). Stress reduction for family caregivers: Effectiveness of adult daycare use. *Journals of Gerontology: Social Sciences, 53B,* S267–S271.

CHAPTER FIFTEEN

Long-Term Care Residences

NATURE AND HISTORY OF LONG-TERM CARE

Long-term care can be provided through in-home services or day care centers. In this chapter, however, the focus is on residential institutions for the elderly. The forms of care provided can range from assistance in dressing, bathing, and ambulating to sophisticated medical life-support systems. The uniqueness of long-term care facilities lies in their constraint on individual choice in everyday situations, as the person living in these settings must adjust to being removed from "normal" individual or family living patterns. Existing long-term care residences include chronic care hospitals, private and public nursing homes, homes for the aged, psychiatric hospitals, and Veterans Administration facilities. All of these facilities provide varied levels of services ranging from extended, skilled, and intermediate care to personal and boarding care. Long-term care facilities are run under a variety of auspices including public, private-nonprofit, or proprietary organizations.

History of Institutional Settings

The history of long-term care institutions in America began with the almshouses and the public poor houses of colonial America. When a family or individual could no longer care for the pauper, that person became the responsibility of the government. The disabled, aged, widowed, orphaned, "feeble-minded" and deranged, and victims of disasters were mixed together in almshouses, hospitals, workhouses, orphanages, and prisons. Officials made little distinction between poverty generated by physical disability and economic distress. Boarding out, or foster care programs, were not uncommon, although often harshly administered (Cohen, 1974). Following the Revolutionary War, almshouses became increasingly popular, and in 1834, the Poor Law of England reaffirmed this approach. The philosophy of isolating the aged and infirm from society continued to be the predominant social policy throughout the nineteenth century.

Residents of almshouses were usually pressed into working for very low wages as a means of earning at least a meager salary. Any financing for the facilities was the responsibility of the towns and counties in which the facilities were located; all efforts at state or federal support were denied for three-quarters of a century. By the late nineteenth century, other resources were being located for some indigent populations, but the elderly were still relegated to the almshouses. In 1875, a New York State report noted:

> Care has been taken not to diminish the terrors of this last resort of poverty, the almshouse, because it has been deemed better that a few should test the minimum rate of which existence can be preserved than that many should find the almshouse so comfortable a home that they would brave the shame of pauperism to gain admission to it. [cited in Cohen, 1974, p. 14]

In the beginning of the twentieth century, the rise of private foundations and philanthropy began to expand the types of institutional care available. In addition, by 1929, the Old Age Assistance Act began to offer an alternative to institutionalization in most states. In the 1930s, new welfare, loan, housing, public works, and rent programs, as well as the Social Security Act (SSA), provided a new concept of income support for the aged.

In the early versions of the SSA, there were prohibitions against federal financial participation in the cost of any relief given in any kind of institutional setting. Later, this prohibition continued in relation to public facilities because public institutions were considered a state responsibility (Cohen, 1974). The intent of the legislation was to encourage the elderly to live at home or with foster families. However, the actual effect was the displacement of people from public facilities—particularly to boarding homes. As these facilities began to add nurses to their staffs, the name "nursing home" emerged (Moss & Halmandaris, 1977). Individuals who could not afford to move to the boarding homes continued in the public homes at state expense (Drake, 1958).

Since the 1930s, the number of institutions providing long-term care has increased rapidly. In 1999, there were 18,000 nursing homes (excluding hospital-based facilities). Federal participation in the cost of assistance for indigent persons in private institutions was first authorized in 1953, but the ban on payment to public institutions continued. However, if states wanted to participate in the federal program, they were required to establish some standards for the institutions. Also, in the 1950s, several federal acts authorized monies through grants and loans for constructing and equipping long-term care institutions. The Hill-Burton Act, the Small Business Administration, and the National Housing Act provisions were the most prominent.

The passage of Medicare in 1965 and Medicaid in 1967 opened new and major funding sources for long-term care institutions. With this legislation, service delivery requirements were reshaped and clarified. Prior to the enactment of Medicare and Medicaid, there was very little consistency among what were defined as institutions of long-term care. Nursing homes, homes for the aged, convalescent hospitals, and chronic care facilities were all defined separately by each state. The new funding sources set common definitions and basic national standards for service delivery in this important area of long-term care (Winston & Wilson, 1977).

Dunlop (1979), however, has argued that the growth in nursing-home beds was greater before passage of Medicaid than after. Indeed, Medicaid replaced earlier forms of medical assistance and has enabled the continuation of nursing-home growth while developing a mechanism for enforcing nursing-home standards.

Extent of Long-Term Care Programs

Despite the extensive increase in the number of long-term care patients, only 4.5% of people aged 65 and over were residents in nursing homes in 2000. Importantly, this percentage is related to age. Although only 1.1% of individuals between the ages of 65 and 74 were living in nursing homes, this figure rises to 18.2% among individuals over the age of 85 (Administration on Aging, 2003). As people get older, their chances of being in a nursing home increase. It is estimated that 43% of all individuals over the age of 65 will spend some time in a nursing home during their lifetime, but for 24% their stay will be less than one year (The Rubins, 2004). In 1999, among all individuals over the age of 65, the average length of stay in nursing homes was 388 days (ElderWeb, n.d., 2000).

Not only has the number of beds increased, but the size of the homes has as well, reflecting the change from family businesses to larger corporations. In 1963, the average nursing home had 39.9 beds; this had increased to 105 beds by 1999 (National Center for Health Statistics, 2002). Nursing homes are primarily for-profit entities (67%) but 27% of the 18,000 homes in the United States in 1999 were under the auspices of nonprofit organizations (National Center for Health Statistics). Large chains such as Beverly Enterprises own more than half of the for-profit nursing homes. In 1997, it was estimated that 3.6 million people would need nursing homes by the year 2018 (National Academy on Aging,

1997). This figure, however, may no longer be accurate because of the growth of other forms of long-term facilities available to older persons and their families. One indicator of the growth of a variety of alternatives to nursing homes was the drop of one percent a year between 1990 and 2000 in the number of nursing home residents in Michigan (Edgar, 2000). Nationally, there was an 11.5% vacancy rate in nursing homes in 2005 (Baker, 2005).

There is an inverse relationship between age and nursing home residency. In 1995, 35% of nursing home residents were over the age of 85, and 90% were over the age of 65. There is only a small representation of minority elderly in nursing homes: 88% of residents are White. As could be expected from life expectancy data, almost three-quarters (72%) of nursing home residents are women (National Center for Health Statistics, 2002).

Importantly, more than 50% of nursing home residents have no living close relatives, which may largely account for the fact that 60% receive no visitors. These figures indicate that one of the contributing factors to nursing home admissions is the lack of family support that might enable the person to continue living in his or her own home.

TYPES OF LONG-TERM CARE RESIDENCES

There are many different types of long-term care facilities for the elderly. However, until the creation of national funding legislation in the mid-1960s, there were no national standards governing the types of care in any given facility. As a result of the Medicare and Medicaid legislation, extended care facilities (ECFs), skilled nursing home services, and intermediate care facilities (ICFs) were identified and defined in terms of standards of care. Since that time, many of the long-term care institutions have adjusted their services to meet the outlined criteria in order to be eligible for reimbursements. Even so, both more extensive care (such as that provided in chronic care hospitals) and less extensive care (such as that provided in assisted living residences) are still under regulation as defined by individual states and, therefore, are more difficult to define nationally.

Assisted Living Residences

Assisted living residences are becoming increasingly popular among more affluent older persons and corporations. In addition to hotel chains that have invested heavily in the development of assisted living complexes, a number of corporations have as their sole business the development and operation of assisted-living complexes. Assisted living has been defined as "a special combination of housing, personalized supportive services and health care, designed to meet the needs—both scheduled and unscheduled—of those who need help with activities of daily living" (Utz, 2003, p. 380). It can also been viewed as a service bridging the gap between living in the community and nursing homes or as an alternative to nursing homes.

Assisted living facilities vary across the U.S. This variation can be seen in the regulations of individual states, the characteristics of the facility, and the managerial experience and training of the staff (Utz, 2003). In general, assisted living facilities provide

- 24-hour assistance with scheduled and unscheduled needs;
- social and recreational activities;
- three meals a day in a dining room;
- laundry, housekeeping, and transportation.

A variety of other amenities may also be available including beauty salons, libraries, and exercise equipment (National Center for Assisted Living, 2001).

In a majority of states, there is still only minimal regulation of assisted living facilities. As regulations impose stricter requirements on these residences, costs may increase. In 2003, the average cost in assisted living facilities was $2,379 per month, an increase of 10% from the previous year. There was wide geographic variation in the average cost: In Washington, D.C., the average cost was $4,429 per month but only $1,020 per month in Jackson, Mississippi. As two-thirds of assisted living residents pay these costs from their own funds, it does not appear that these facilities are an option for lower-income elderly. Despite the high costs, the growth in the number of these facilities has been steady. Between 1998 and 2003, the number of assisted living facilities grew by 48% to a total of 36,999 communities (The rising cost of assisted living, 2003).

As assisted living facilities increase in number, there is concern about the quality of care that they provide. Regulations have been proposed that would prevent small hotels or board and care residences from calling themselves "assisted living." Data from assisted living facilities indicate that their residents clearly need a range of help. Among residents living in these facilities in 2000, 30% used a walker, and 15% a wheelchair. Whereas 27% of the residents need help with 4–5 of the activities of daily living, only 19% could carry out these activities by themselves. Approximately three-quarters of the residents require some assistance with the "instrumental activities of daily living" such as transportation, shopping, taking their medications and managing their money (National Center for Assisted Living, 2001). The withdrawal of some hotel chains from this market indicates that there may be some overbuilding of these facilities or that it is becoming increasingly difficult to make a profit and still provide the services that residents of these facilities need.

In October 2004, New York enacted new regulations for assisted living residences. These regulations resulted from injuries or deaths at several facilities. The state health department must now license assisted living facilities in New York. The range of services that they must provide is defined. Requirements are most stringent for facilities that want to accept incontinent patients, non-ambulatory residents, or dementia patients. Service plans must be developed for each resident and updated every six months. Residences must be inspected every 18 months for violations (AARP, 2004).

Skilled Nursing Facilities

> Skilled nursing facilities are required to provide certain services, including the emergency and ongoing services of a physician, nursing care, rehabilitative services, pharmaceutical services, dietetic services, laboratory and radiologic services, dental services, social services, and activity services. [Glasscote et al., 1976, p. 34]

Some of these services must be a part of the facility itself, but rehabilitative, laboratory, radiological, social, and dental services may be provided by formal contractual agreement with outside resources.

There must be visits by attending physicians every 30 days of the first 90 days of a patient's stay. After that time, if justified, the visits can be reduced to every 60 days. A patient care plan should also be prepared and reviewed regularly, so that the patient is assured of receiving services that are needed, and changing conditions are translated into appropriate care.

In 1986, a report of the National Institute of Medicine criticized the quality of care and life in nursing homes. The report stressed the need for greater federal involvement in the regulation of nursing home operation. In 1987, new federal rules were passed in Congress that strengthened inspection of nursing homes accepting Medicare or Medicaid funds. Although the states can waive the rules in some cases, these homes must have a registered nurse on duty at least 8 hours each day and a licensed practical nurse on duty at all times. A social worker with a bachelor's degree in social work is required at all homes of over 120 beds. In addition, new training requirements for aides were instituted. Regular programs of activities, use and preparation of drugs, and physical facilities in relation to fire and safety codes are carefully delineated for skilled nursing facilities. In general, skilled nursing facilities can be characterized as medical institutions that care for patients who are severely ill. The most recent development in skilled nursing home care is the growth of separate units within existing homes, or even separate nursing homes, for Alzheimer's disease patients. These "special-care units" began in the 1980s. By the mid-1990s, 15% of nursing homes now had special care units that provided 50,000 beds to older persons with Alzheimer's disease or related disorders. These units varied in size, staff, auspices and programs (Advisory Panel on Alzheimer's Disease, 1996).

This diversity provides options for patients and their families; however, it has made evaluation of the effectiveness of the program difficult. Although it may be easier for staff to care for residents in these specialized settings, research does not indicate that special care units improve their functioning (Chappell & Reid, 2000).

Another alternative model attempts to develop nursing homes that are smaller and more personal in orientation than the large multi-bed facilities that are now predominant. Termed the "Green House Project," these nursing homes focus on a model that stresses the social environment. The homes aim for about 10 resident with private bedrooms centered around a common area. The first Green Houses opened in Tupelo, Mississippi, in 2003 (Baker, 2005).

Intermediate Care Facilities

Intermediate care facilities (ICFs) were defined in conjunction with the Medicaid legislation of the late 1960s. The definition evolved from the recognition that a large number of poor people were not ill enough to require full-time professional staff attention, but did need health supervision and access to various health and rehabilitative components (Glasscote et al., 1976). This level of care is defined only in terms of Medicaid reimbursement. Those patients who are paying privately pay a fee established by the nursing home, and are not involved in the definitions of levels of care.

Intermediate care can be provided not only in facilities that are set up for that purpose, but in skilled care facilities, homes for the aged, hospitals, or personal care homes. In other words, as with skilled care, the definition of intermediate care lies in the level of care provided, rather than in the facility providing that care.

Many regulations are the same as for skilled nursing facilities:

> Regulations for construction, sanitation, safety, and the handling of drugs are very similar. Theoretically and philosophically the difference is that the SNF is a "medical" institution and the ICF is a "health" institution. In the ICF, social and recreational policy is to be given near equal emphasis with medical policy. [Glasscote et al., 1976, p. 39]

In addition, there are lesser requirements for supervisory personnel. For example, on the day shift, either a registered nurse or a licensed practical nurse must supervise nursing services. This is a less sophisticated nursing requirement than that of the skilled nursing facility.

The federal regulations for both skilled nursing facilities and ICFs leave room for interpretation, new regulations, and elaboration. This is important, because it allows the states who administer, supervise, and control the nursing home program to build an improved program based on their own particular needs and resources. It is also the states that set the criteria of who is eligible for which level of care. Potential patients who are eligible for Medicare must have their conditions reviewed by the locally designated authority to determine the appropriate level of care for each condition. The nursing home is then reimbursed for the designated level of care, with the intermediate level determination receiving less reimbursement than the skilled level. The levels of care must be separated, either by facility or by wings in a facility. Because of this requirement, if the condition of a patient already admitted to a nursing home should change to the extent that the required level of care changes, that patient will either be moved to another section of the nursing home or, in some cases, be moved to another facility. A private paying patient who becomes eligible for Medicaid after admission will, at that time, be evaluated and assigned a level of care that might or might not require a physical change.

Mental Hospitals

Mental hospitals continue to care for the elderly, but not in as significant numbers as before. Many of the older patients are among the long-term hospital population. Large numbers of older individuals were transferred out of state mental hospitals following the passage of Medicare and Medicaid legislation. Many of these former state hospital patients instead became residents of nursing homes. The number of older patients in state hospitals has also been restricted by decisions in state and federal courts, which have made grounds for involuntary commitment to mental hospitals much more stringent. In 1999, the number of patients in state mental hospital was less than 100,000. Even ignoring the growth of the U.S. population, this figure represents a tremendous reduction from the 550,000 individuals who were living in these facilities 50 years earlier (Eisenberg, 1999).

Since 1989, the federal government has attempted to restrict the use of nursing homes as substitutes for mental hospitals. At present, nursing facilities may not admit persons with mental illness or retardation to a nursing home unless they are first evaluated by the state to determine whether they need the services of a nursing home and active mental health treatment. Once admitted to a nursing home, the resident's condition must be reviewed annually to assess if he or she still needs to be in the nursing home and requires active mental health treatment. If the answer on these two criteria is negative, the resident must be discharged from the nursing home. Anyone who has resided in the nursing home for more than 30 months has the choice to stay in the facility or move to another setting. The state must also provide treatment for those individuals in the nursing home whose assessment indicates it is needed. Importantly, Alzheimer's disease and dementia are not considered mental illnesses under Pre-Admission and Annual Resident Review. If this assessment and review process is enforced and substantial numbers of older persons are either kept out of nursing homes and hospitals or are discharged, there may be problems related to finding appropriate placements for them (Jones & Kamter, 1989).

FUNDING

The funding system of long-term care facilities has been a major influence on the development of types of facilities and care that are available. The two most important sources, in terms of shaping the long-term care industry, are Medicare and Medicaid. As indicated earlier, Medicare legislation, which was passed in 1965, authorized care in a long-term care institution for those patients who were hospitalized for at least 3 consecutive days, who needed skilled nursing care, and who were to be admitted to a Medicare-certified facility within 14 days of their discharge from the hospital. The patient had to be evaluated regularly and could stay in the long-term care facility for no longer than 90 days under Medicare.

In 1969, the rapidly rising costs for the program led to a change in the regulations. New administrative regulations required that participants in the program have rehabilitative potential. In addition, nursing care was defined in more narrow terms, which included only a very limited number of diagnoses and therapeutic situations. The effect of these new regulations was to virtually cut off Medicare as a vehicle for nursing home care for the elderly (Moss & Halmandaris, 1977). Because many nursing homes were caught losing thousands of dollars in disallowed costs at the time the regulations changed, the number of nursing homes that wanted to participate in the Medicare program dramatically decreased. However, the precedent of reimbursement for medical long-term care was set.

Legislation establishing Medicaid—a system of medical cost reimbursement for the poor—opened the greatest opportunity for funding nursing home care. In 2000, Medicaid expenditures for nursing home care amounted to $44 billion. In comparison, Medicare spent $9 billion for nursing home care in 1980 (Centers for Medicare & Medicaid Services, n.d.). Because Medicaid is a shared federal-state program, the federal government provides a basic set of requirements upon which the states build the program. The states determine their own definitions of "needy"; there is some flexibility from state to state as to who is eligible for Medicaid in long-term care institutions. States can include the categorically needy (those who are eligible for federally aided financial assistance) and the medically needy (those whose incomes are sufficient for daily living expenses, but are not enough to pay for medical expenses). Because of the nature of this definition, persons who might not be eligible while in the community could be eligible for Medicaid if entering a long-term care residence. Often, the residential Medicaid eligibility factors for long-term care residences relate more to personal assets than monthly income, and so once the assets are liquidated, a person entering a nursing home can become eligible for Medicaid reimbursements.

Formerly, to achieve eligibility, a married couple had to "spend down" almost all of their assets. One result was that the spouse who remained living in the community was reduced to impoverished conditions. Under the "spousal impoverishment" provisions of Medicaid, the spouse remaining in the community is now allowed to retain a maximum of up to one-half of the couple's assets and a minimum of $18,132 (in 2003). The states are allowed to raise this minimum. By 1991, some states had raised the minimum to the maximum, a change that allows the older couple to preserve a good portion of their assets. The maximum in 2005 was $95,100 (Illinois Department of Insurance, 2005). The couple's house can be transferred to the community-based spouse without penalty. Other possible transferees include minor, blind, or disabled children living in the house or sons or daughters who lived in the home for 2 years as a caregiver prior to the institutionalization of the nursing home resident. Residents can also enter a home as private paying patients, and as their assets diminish, they become eligible for Medicaid.

Extensive publicity has been generated about potential abuses of Medicaid reimbursements. As Moss and Halmandaris (1977) point out, conflicts between profits and quality of care are likely when services become a money-making operation. The conflicts will be greatest in firms that operate a number of homes, as they may attempt to maximize their profits by lowering the costs they incur at any one particular home. State regulatory agencies, understanding the financial incentives of the nursing home industry, promulgate reimbursement regulations that are designed to encourage quality care and limit profits. There have been variations in the success of these regulations.

Under the Medicaid program, nursing homes are reimbursed in relation to their costs. All costs must be included in the reimbursement fee, and the patient is not to be charged extra for services given. The states must set their reimbursement rates to allow the nursing homes to operate efficiently and meet quality standards. In setting their cost rates, the states are also expected to take into account the special situation of nursing homes that predominantly serve low-income individuals. Medicare also uses a cost-related system for reimbursement, but allows a prospective reimbursement for some types of nursing homes.

All patients in nursing homes under Medicaid are eligible for at least $30 a month in spending money for anything the patient wants, including cigarettes, haircuts, clothes, and magazines. This spending money is in exchange for the fact that any income the patient is receiving, such as Social Security, is to be paid to the home and subtracted from the amount of the Medicaid reimbursement. For those patients who can personally handle the money, the program is successful. However, for those patients who cannot manage their own resources, there has been potential for abuse in the use of the money, as it can come under the supervision of the nursing home administration.

Private Payments

As already noted, a significant percentage of nursing home payments come directly from the patients or their families. A patient may have significant assets and enter the institution as a private paying resident. At an average cost of $181 per day in 2003 for skilled nursing care, payments can quickly deplete all of a resident's assets (Met Life Mature Market News, 2003). In 2001, 46% of all nursing home costs were paid by Medicaid (Federal Interagency Forum on Aging Related Statistics, 2004). Although Medicaid places restrictions on the charges for nursing home care, individuals who are privately paying for the nursing home can be charged for extra services that may be required for care. For example, extra bed padding, extra toileting time, and extra time for feeding could all result in additional charges. Private paying patients usually cannot predict the exact costs of the home, and have no recourse if they object to the prices charged except to find another nursing home. As these costs of nursing home care mount up over time, long-term residents and their families may be forced to evaluate whether they are eligible for Medicaid coverage of these costs.

The Green Homes provide staffing that is double that of most nursing homes. However, proponents claim that these homes result in cost savings because of the coordination of services staff members provide. This coordination allows for the elimination of separate departments for housekeeping, dietary, and personal care services. In addition, the initial results that indicate better health and emotional functioning of residents can result in reduced reliance on such items as food supplements and products for incontinence. Most importantly in terms of cost is that staff turnover is greatly reduced (Baker, 2005).

Much of the care that is provided under board and care, personal care, and domiciliary care homes is paid directly by the residents of the facilities. SSI and Social Security checks are turned over to the facility in exchange for personal care services that are rendered.

Long-term care insurance that covers skilled nursing home and in-home care is now offered through many private insurers. The number and purchasers of these policies increased dramatically during the last part of the 1980s. Although only 17 companies offered long-term care insurance before 1985, this number had grown to 130 by 1991 (Moon & Mulvey, 1995). In 2000, 4 million U.S. residents were purchasing long-term care insurance (Merlis, 2003). There have been strong criticisms of many of the policies offered because their benefits are inadequate and they do not adjust for inflation. Without an inflation clause, the policy may continue to reimburse $100 per day for nursing home care in 2006 and the same $100 per day in 2020, when nursing home costs may have risen substantially. Many policies have also contained clauses excluding individuals with preexisting conditions.

The policies allow the individual to choose a nursing home benefit, usually $100 or $200 a day. For nursing home care, the whole benefit is paid. For home health care, adult day care, and homemaker services such as meal preparation, laundry, and shopping, one-half of the daily benefit is paid. Some policies will also pay for respite care, including a stay by the patient in a custodial care facility or a visit from a companion who serves as a substitute caregiver. An assessment that the individual had a preexisting condition 6 months before enrolling in the plan could delay payment of benefits for 6 months. The individual must demonstrate that he or she is unable to perform two of the activities of daily living before becoming eligible for benefits. According to the Health Insurance Association of America, the cost of a long-term care policy for a healthy 65-year-old individual is about $3,000 per year (Brooks, 1996).

Long-term care insurance remains a new, important, but basically untested approach to long-term care. The expensive payments may deter many 65-year-old persons from enrolling. A 2003 study indicates that three-quarters of couples below the age of 59 could afford long-term care insurance (Merlis, 2003). Even lower costs of approximately $1,500 per year may seem high to the 55-year-old who cannot envision the future need for this type of benefit. The benefits for home care may also not be sufficient to meet the needs of severely impaired elderly who do not have relatives or friends nearby to supplement the care provided by a home health aide or nurse.

A major investment firm advises that individuals may want long-term care insurance if they have a family history of major medical problems and can afford the premiums. However, they suggest that this form of insurance may not be worthwhile if net worth is below $500,000 or over $1.5 million, or the individual is paying the large premiums required if this insurance is bought at a later age (Fidelity Retirement, 2004).

A policy bought in 2005 by a 50-year-old individual may also not take into account the future "financing environment" in long-term care:

> That environment could change in any number of ways, making a specific policy obsolete. There are likely to be further efforts to develop prepaid systems that integrate acute and long-term care. There may be newer forms of supportive housing arrangements. New technologies might reduce the needs for hands-on care for some kinds of patients. Medicare benefits might be modified, to cover more or fewer long-term care services, or some new public financing program for long-term care might be adopted—potentially overlapping with coverage under private LTCI [Long-Term Care Insurance] policies. Any of these changes could mean that a policy bought today could have less value in the future or could fail to provide access to newly emerging service options. [Merlis, 2003, p. vi]

The overall conclusion is that "Stand-alone LTCI products are a sensible investment for only a small minority of active workers" (Merlis, 2003, p. vi). The validity of this controversial assertion will be only become clear over time.

A combination of public and private long-term insurance may become more prevalent in future decades. A plan adopted in New York and a number of other states allows individuals who purchase long-term care insurance to keep a dollar in assets for each dollar of insurance they purchase. This proviso reduces the assets that must be spent to qualify for Medicaid. The equity of this type of plan for older people of different incomes has been contested as well as its ability to adequately pay for nursing home care (estimated at $62,000 per year in New York) (Freudenheim, 1992).

State and Local Funding

State funding, which covers about one-half of the Medicaid reimbursement (it varies slightly from state to state), reimburses the board and care, personal care, and domiciliary care facilities when personal income is inadequate to cover the allowed daily reimbursement rate. It also covers the costs of individual care in mental hospitals, and in these settings the total cost of patient care is paid. One of the reasons for the increase in the number of elderly who are being transferred to nursing homes and personal care facilities from state hospitals is the states' desire to develop a situation where the federal government is paying at least part of the cost of caring for the elderly.

Long-term care facilities provide an excellent example of how the funding mechanisms have shaped the types and amount of services available for the elderly. In addition, long-term care is unique in that the majority of care is being provided by profit-making organizations, a factor that both influences and is influenced by the funding available for this particular type of service. Whatever the source, the cost of nursing home care is striking.

PERSONNEL AND PROGRAMMING

Staffing Patterns

Staffing patterns of long-term care residences are closely related to reimbursement rates. Homes attempt to meet state regulations regarding personnel while at the same time keeping costs in line with reimbursement allowances, including profit. Unfortunately, the end result is generally an inadequate and poorly trained staff. Aides and orderlies perform between 80% and 90% of all nursing care actually given patients. Most aides and orderlies receive no training for their jobs, and high turnover rates among these important personnel remain a problem. One major reason for the lack of trained and committed staff is the salary, which is usually at or just above minimum wage. This is a disincentive to produce a commitment to the job, to seek additional training, or even to stay on the job for any length of time beyond that of getting enough experience to get another, perhaps better-paying, job. However, any job training beyond the minimal in-service programs required by the homes would raise the demands for higher wages, which in turn would reflect directly on the Medicaid reimbursement figures. Community colleges are beginning to offer special training for aides, which in certain situations could help provide stability to staffing patterns.

In contrast to the prevailing pattern in most nursing homes, Green Home Projects rely on a trained certified nurse's aide (termed a "shahbaz") to coordinate services for residents. These aides have received an additional 200 hours of first aid, cooking, and counseling skills and are supported by nurses and therapists (Baker, 2005).

The number of staff (including aides) actually on the floor of a nursing home influences the quality and amount of care given. The stated minimum requirement, which varies from state to state, usually says that a certain amount (2 to 3 hours) of nursing care is required per patient per day. However, when this is translated to personnel, it could be actual on-floor nursing care, or on-floor care except for lunches and breaks, absences, and vacations. For the latter, the actual on-floor care is half an hour below that required. The interpretation affects the care, the cost, the reimbursement rate, and the profit margin. Some states have been reluctant to interpret such regulations precisely until they can generate a Medicaid reimbursement rate that can pay for actual staffing requirements.

In addition to the basic nursing and support staff, homes are required to have access to certain types of professional staff. The extent to which the home actually hires the professional person required, as opposed to responding to the need through contractual agreements, affects the quality of care in the home. For example, actually hiring a social worker, a dietitian, an occupational therapist, and a full-time physician brings more services to the home than using these people a few hours a week on a contract basis. The size of the home, whether the home is part of a larger chain of homes (the individual hired by a chain of homes can work in two or three facilities), and the type of reimbursement mechanism influence the extent to which the home actually hires the additional personnel required.

Programming and Advocacy

Beyond having an activity director whose responsibility is to provide some activity for patients, state regulations do not stipulate the types of programming for nursing homes. The result is that there is a tremendous variety of programmed activities available in long-term care institutions. Some homes make only the minimum number of programs available, whereas others establish links with the community to ensure that those programs most appropriate to the patients' needs are presented.

Sensory training, reality orientation, and remotivation are essential components of nursing home programming. Reorientation of patients to the larger world, heightening their sensory sensitivity, and reestablishing earlier interests all help to improve their daily functioning. As in other major services, the range of activities that may be well received by patients runs the gamut from picnics, dance, theater, and crafts to movies and guest speakers. Some nursing homes have links with senior centers, adult day care centers, and nutrition programs in order to provide ways of getting patients into other settings and of bringing community people into the nursing homes. Volunteer organizations from the community also provide special services for patients in many community nursing homes.

Programming that has a purpose and revitalizes the interests and talents of the patients are the most successful. Many patients have little opportunity to share their experiences and even themselves with others when they enter a nursing home. Programming can create these opportunities if patients see it as meaningful. Families can also be built into the programming for the home. However, if a patient has only minimal family ties, the nursing home can create an atmosphere of the extended family by bringing in friendly visiting volunteers and using other patients, when appropriate.

Two advocacy programs in recent years have focused on the special needs of patients in long-term care settings, particularly nursing homes, and on how to get those needs vocalized in a way that produces a response. One, the patients' rights movement, began in the early 1970s when several states passed patients' rights legislation in response to the belief that the personal rights and liberties of patients were being lost with the institutional process (Wilson, 1978). In 1974, the federal government developed regulations that established a set of rights for patients in skilled and intermediate care facilities. These rights, which relate to individual liberties and dignities, must be readily displayed, explained to the patients, and assigned to nursing home personnel for enforcement. Some of the rights covered in the regulations include

- being informed of the services available in the facility
- being informed of one's medical condition and the plan of treatment
- being encouraged and assisted throughout the stay in the nursing home
- being able to manage personal financial affairs
- being free from mental and physical abuse
- being assured of confidential treatment of personal and medical records
- being able to retain use of personal clothing and possessions as space permits
- being assured privacy for visits by one's spouse

Unfortunately, there are conditional clauses that make enforcement difficult, and the only disciplinary tool available is decertification of the facility, a recourse that is too severe for individual violations.

The second advocacy program created to respond to specific needs of patients is the ombudsman program, which is designed to examine complaints by patients and, through investigations, give them a voice in determining their own circumstances. Begun in 1972, five ombudsman programs were funded nationally as models of the ways that the program could be most effective. Two more programs were added in 1973. Today, most ombudsman programs are affiliated with the State Units on Aging and work through the Area Agencies on Aging. They still retain the objective of being the focal point for complaints regarding nursing home care, but they also act as a nursing home referral service, an organizer of friendly visiting programs, and a center for educating patients and the community on the rights of nursing home patients (Administration on Aging, 1977).

In recent years, the role of the ombudsman has been strengthened through both federal and state legislation. The nursing home reforms place an emphasis on nursing home residents knowing about the ombudsman program. In New Jersey the state ombudsman is permitted to investigate complaints and hold hearings as well as subpoena individuals and records. In the District of Columbia the ombudsman serves as "resident's representative" and can file petitions for receivership, as well as complaints for civil damages and actions against the District (Schuster, 1989).

Title VII of the 1992 OAA amendments defined the functions and duties of the ombudsman more extensively than in the 1987 amendments. The functions range from investigation of complaints to informing residents of long-term care facilities, means of obtaining services, and ensuring that the residents obtain these services. The duties are similar to the functions, but also include review and comment on proposed laws and regulations that may affect residents, facilitation of public access to review of these laws and regulations, and support for the development of resident and family councils in long-term care residences.

The number of complaints investigated by ombudsmen rose from 145,000 in 1996 to 186,000 in 2000 (Health and Human Services Office of the Inspector General, 2000) and to 261,000 in 2002. The ombudsman programs relied on 8,000 volunteers working through local agencies, most of which were area agencies on aging (National Association of State Units on Aging, 2004). Despite the rise in the number of complaints, there has been no change in the major types of complaints. The top six categories included (1) failure to respond to a call for assistance, (2) accusations of improper handling of a patient, (3) lack of an adequate patient care plan. (4) inadequate administration of medication, (5) unattended resident symptoms, and (6) poor personal hygiene of the patient (Health and Human Services Office of the Inspector General, 2000).

QUALITY IN LONG-TERM CARE RESIDENCES

How well the long-term-care residence is carrying out its mandate, meeting requirements, and providing the level of care agreed to under its contract with the funding sources is evaluated through the inspection system. The federal government provides the regulative substructure on which the states build specific codes for operation. The states then divide the inspection responsibilities between local fire and safety agencies. The result is a series of inspections of the homes for different purposes, which are, at times, in conflict with one another.

The two biggest problems with the current inspection systems are that (1) inspections are primarily to evaluate the physical plant rather than the actual quality of care because actual quality of care is very difficult to measure, long lists of physical requirements become the substitute, and (2) there is essentially no weapon for noncompliance except revoking the license to operate—a very difficult step, in many cases inappropriate to the situation, both because the need for nursing home beds is so acute and because shutting down a home and moving patients is traumatic; hence, a state or local enforcement body will not usually impose such a step until after years of flagrant abuse.

Basically, most states have four components to their inspection systems: (1) sanitation and environment, (2) meals, (3) fire safety, and (4) patient care. This means that there is a visit by a sanitarian, a dietitian, a professional review team, and a fire inspector (Moss & Halmandaris, 1977). In most states, at least two of the inspections are to be unannounced, although this is not always the case. Until the inspection system develops better organized procedures and more effective ways of measuring the actual quality of care, this system will not be the best answer to improving the care in long-term care residences. Between 2000 and 2003, the number of nursing homes cited for violating federal standards declined 18% (Pear, 2004). It is unclear, however, whether this decline resulted from improved performance of the homes or less vigorous enforcement of standards by inspectors.

In 1987, a comprehensive set of nursing home reform amendments was passed, which went into effect in October 1990. Under the amendments, skilled nursing facilities and intermediate care facilities are termed "nursing facilities" and are held to a single standard of care. Within each of these facilities, a comprehensive assessment of residents must be undertaken at admission, when the residents' physical or mental condition changes, and at least on an annual basis. These assessments form the basis of a care plan designed to help the residents maintain or attain the highest level of physical, mental, and psychosocial functioning possible given their condition.

Each facility must have a licensed nurse on duty at all times. A registered nurse must be on duty during at least one shift per day. The nurse aides who work at the nursing facilities must complete a 75-hour training course within 4 months of being hired. A physician must visit the home every 30 days during the first 3 months of a resident's stay and thereafter every 90 days. The amendments allow the visits to be conducted by a physician's assistant or nurse practitioner, if supervised by a physician. A full-time social worker must also be employed in all nursing facilities over 120 beds in size.

All of the above changes are an effort to ensure quality of care in nursing facilities. In addition, the facilities must maintain a Quality Assessment and Assurance Committee that can identify the issues that need to be assessed and implement action designed to correct deficiencies. The facility must also offer an activities program and rehabilitative services. An independent consultant must be utilized to monitor all psychopharmacologic drugs. The amendments also include a clear statement of residents' rights in the home (National Citizen's Coalition for Nursing Home Reform, n.d.).

REFERENCES

AARP. (2004, December). AARP nation: New York gets tough on assisted living laws. *AARP Bulletin, 49*, 23.

Administration on Aging. (1977). *Nursing home ombudsman program: A fact sheet and program directory.* Washington, DC: U.S. Government Printing Office.

Administration on Aging. (2003). *A profile of older Americans: 2003.* Retrieved November 5, 2004 from http://research.aarp.org/general/profile_2003.pdf

Advisory Panel on Alzheimer's Disease. (1996). *Alzheimer's disease and related dementias: Report to Congress.* Washington, DC: U.S. Government Printing Office.Assisted living continues to be hot issue, AAHA says. (1993). *Older American Reports, 17*, 259.

Baker, B. (2005). Small world. *AARP Bulletin, 46*(9), 28–29, 39.

Brooks, A. (1996, August 15). Pitfalls in home-care insurance for the elderly. *New York Times*, p. B4.

Centers for Medicare & Medicaid Services, Office of the Actuary, National Health Statistics Group; U.S. Bureau of the Census. (n.d.). Retrieved June 3, 2005, from http://www.efmoody.com/longterm/nursingstatistics.html

Chappell, N., & Reid, B. (2000). Dimensions of care for dementia sufferers in long-term care institutions: Are they related to outcomes? *Journals of Gerontology: Social Sciences, 55*, S234–S244.

Cohen, E. (1974). An overview of long-term care facilities. In E. Brody (Ed.), *A social work guide for long-term care facilities* (pp. 11–26). Rockville, MD: National Institute of Mental Health.

Drake, J. (1958). *The aged in American society.* New York: Ronald.

Dunlop, B. (1979). *The growth of nursing home care.* Lexington, MA: Lexington Books.

Edgar, J. (2000, November 16). Nursing homes seek revival: Assisted living's extra comforts claiming clients. *Detroit Free Press*, p. 1B.

Eisenberg, L. (1999). The limits of prediction: The future ain't what it used to be. *American Journal of Psychiatry, 156*, 501–503.

ElderWeb. (n.d.). *Housing and care: Nursing homes.* Retrieved November 1, 2004, from http://www.elderweb.com/default.php?PageID=2770

Federal Interagency Forum on Aging Related Statistics. (2004). *Sources of payment for health care services.* Retrieved December 21, 2004, from http://www.agingstats.gov/chartbook2004/healthcare.html#Indicator%2033

Fidelity Retirement. (2004). *Relief from the burden of long-term care.* October, 10–11.

Freudenheim, M. (1992, May 3). Medicaid plan promotes nursing-home insurance. *New York Times,* pp. 1, 20.

Glasscote, R., Biegel, A., Jr., Clark, E., Cox, B., Wiper, J. R., Gudeman, J. E. et al. (1976). *Old folks at homes.* Washington, DC: American Psychiatric Association and the Mental Health Association.

Health and Human Services Office of the Inspector General. (2000). *State ombudsman data: Nursing home complaints.* Retrieved August 30, 2004, from http://www.oig.hhs.gov/reports/oei-09-02-00160.pdf

Illinois Department of Insurance. (2005). *Spousal impoverishment.* Retrieved June 8, 2005, from http://www.idfpr.com/DOI/Ship/spousal_impov.asp

Jones, E., & Kamter, A. (1989). Advocating for freedom: The community placement of elders from state psychiatric hospitals. *Clearinghouse Review, 44,* 444–449.

Merlis, M. (2003). *Private long-term care insurance: Who should buy it and what should they buy?* Retrieved February 10, 2005, from http://www.kff.org

Met Life Mature Market News. *Mature Market News.* (2003). Retrieved June 3, 2005, from http://www.ltcadvisers.com/2003NursingHomeCosts.htm

Moon, M., & Mulvey, J. (1995). *Entitlements and the elderly: Protecting promises, recognizing realities.* Washington, DC: Urban Institute Press.

Moss, F., & Halmandaris, V. (1977). *Too old, too sick, too bad.* Germantown, MD: Aspen Systems Group.

National Academy on Aging. (1997). *Facts on long-term care.* Washington, DC: Author.

National Association of State Units on Aging. (2004). *Long-term care ombudsman program.* Retrieved November 9, 2004, from http://www.nasua.org/elderrights/ombudsman.htm

National Center for Assisted Living. (2001). *Facts and figures: Assisted living sourcebook.* Retrieved October 25, 2004, from http://www.anca.org/research/alsourcebook2001.pdf

National Center for Health Statistics. (2002). *1999 summary. Data from the 1999 National Nursing Home Survey.* Hyattsville, MD: Author.

National Citizen's Coalition for Nursing Home Reform. (n.d.). *A brief summary of selected key provisions of the Nursing Home Reform Amendments of OBRA '87.* Washington, DC: Author.

Pear, R. (2004, August 8). Penalties for nursing homes show a drop in last 4 years. *New York Times,* p. A11.

The rising cost of assisted living. (2003, October 26). *New York Times,* 3:8.

The Rubins. (2004). *Statistics on nursing homes and their residents.* Retrieved November 6, 2004, from http://www.therubins.com/homes/stathome.htm

Schuster, M. (1989). Legal support to the long-term care ombudsman program: A practical guide. *Clearinghouse Review, 44,* 418–421.

Utz, R. (2003). Assisted living: The philosophical challenges of everyday practice. *Journal of Applied Gerontology, 22,* 379–404.

Wilson, S. (1978). Nursing home patients' rights: Are they enforceable? *The Gerontologist, 18,* 255–261.

Winston, W., & Wilson, A. (1977). *Ethical considerations in long-term care.* St. Petersburg, FL: Eckerd College Gerontology Center.

CHAPTER SIXTEEN

Challenges for the Aging Network

The latter part of the 20th century saw an enormous growth in the number and quality of programs and services oriented to older Americans. There are at least three questions that now must be faced: (1) Are these programs and services adequate and equitable? (2) Will they be able to respond to new demands in the 21st century? (3) Will they be financed by government, older people and their families, or some combination of these?

There is little doubt that the first part of the twenty-first century will see a slow but steady increase in the number of older people. This growth rate will accelerate as the "baby boomers" born between 1946 and 1963 move into their later years. There is a lot of commentary about the size of this group. As important as its size are the characteristics of this age cohort.

In 1946, returning veterans of World War II embraced the living opportunities held out by the new American suburbs and moved with their young families to these communities. They purchased homes and automobiles and developed a life style that is still pervasive in the United States. If the veterans themselves did not attend college, many of them believed that education was important for their children. Mass higher education became a norm.

In the 1970s with the rise of the feminist movement, women began not only to attend college in large numbers but to set their sights on careers that were outside the four major professions formerly seen as appropriate for women: social work, librarianship, nursing, and teaching.

Many social welfare programs maintain a social problem orientation: that is, a problem exists and efforts need to be developed that target and reduce the negative effects of this problem. As has been argued vociferously over the past 30 years, aging is not a problem. It is a natural process that unfortunately was not allowed to take place in many societies. Mortality rates among infants and young children prevented individuals from reaching later stages of life. These later stages can be very positive or negative in their impact. What is clear, however, is that increasing numbers of individuals in developing and developed societies will encounter the later stages of life. In developed societies such as the United States, these later stages may take on profiles that were not even contemplated at the turn of the century. This can be seen by a brief examination of the possible life course of Americans in the 21st century.

For many Americans, school has become an extended period of life. Where high school was an educational endpoint for most individuals in 1950, it is increasingly seen as a terminal that restricts employment opportunities unless followed by a college education. Even a bachelor's degree, however, is now seen as an entry level for many professions. Increasingly, graduate education is required for advancement in fields that include business, law, academia, the health professions, and social welfare. With this emphasis, it is not surprising to find many individuals remaining in school until they are 25.

After this long period of education, individuals enter into their years of employment. Until the 1980s, it was assumed that retirement occurred at age 65. This expectation is no longer correct as the proportion of workers retiring at earlier ages continues to increase. Many workers are now retiring as early as age 55, often encouraged by "buy-outs" from companies interested in replacing higher-paid, older workers with lower-paid new employees. The old phrase of "30 years and out" may thus still be true for many workers.

Having retired at age 55, the individual may now enter a period of retirement that lasts 30 years. This estimate is based on the life expectancy of those reaching the age of 65. In 2000, women could expect to live an additional 19.3 years on average, and men an additional 16.2 years (National Center for Health Statistics, 2003). The possibility thus now exists that the longest period of a person's life may be that time when he or she no longer faces work responsibilities. How to utilize this extended period beyond "killing time" is one of the challenges that will face many older Americans. As the stage of school expands at one end of the life cycle and retirement at the other, programs and services will have an important role to play in meeting this new opportunity and challenge.

POPULATION GROWTH

A social problems approach to aging cannot confront the implications of the growth of the older population. This growth means that the society has been able to mitigate many of the basic negative conditions related to poor environment and health that make it impossible for many people to enjoy their later years. That these positive changes can also be reversed is indicated by the substantial reduction in life expectancy that has occurred in Russia in recent years.

The challenge for programs and services is twofold: (1) to enable older people to maintain their health and social functioning and engage in activities that they find rewarding, and (2) to enable them to enter their later years with adequate financial resources.

The first challenge is one to which all service providers probably subscribe. The second is more difficult. Even if this is one of their goals, services targeted at older people can only hope to remedy or alleviate problems encountered by people at younger ages. These problems may be the result of a whole set of inadequate services available in the community. They may also result from major structural issues such as restricted job opportunities, discrimination, or inadequate educational systems. Statistics such as the high proportion of high school dropouts among Latino students have negative implications for the health and economic status of future Latino cohorts of elderly. Problems in later life may also stem from the failure of individuals to engage in a healthy lifestyle, including adequate diet and exercise.

INCREASING DIVERSITY

The United States of the 1960s was a country of White descendants of European stock. Added to this group was a substantial population of Black residents with African roots, Native Americans whose numbers had been depleted through almost two centuries of warfare and impoverishment, Latino residents whose roots could often be traced to periods before the annexation of the Southwest into the United States, and a small population of Asians, predominantly from Japanese and Chinese backgrounds.

The United States in 2006 was considerably different than the United States of 1960. The Latino population is rapidly growing through immigration and a high birth rate. Latinos are now the largest minority population in the United States, coming from a variety of countries in Latin America with a diversity of cultural backgrounds and beliefs. The African American population continues to grow, but not as rapidly as the Latino.

The Asian population is also growing rapidly, and is very visible in its concentration in a number of urban areas. This population growth, spurred on by immigration reform of 1965 and the end of the Vietnam War, now includes not only substantial numbers of Chinese and Japanese but also Vietnamese, Cambodians, Laotians, Filipinos, Indians, and

Koreans. Political conditions in countries such as Haiti have also promoted immigration to the United States. Political problems in other areas of the world, including Eastern Europe and Hong Kong, promise to continue the United States' role as the destination of choice of individuals suffering economic or political problems.

For some Americans, the changed political composition of the country appears threatening to basic values and economic opportunities. For others, it presents a new challenge: how to utilize the vitality of new cultural infusions into a country whose cultural institutions reflect a variety of European influences. Whatever our views on diversity may be, the backgrounds of future cohorts of elderly will be much more varied than they have been in the past. Some of the seniors who will be served in coming decades arrived in the United States as adults of various ages. Others arrived as children. Some will speak English fluently; others will not. Some will have strong connections to family in this country. In other cases, families will have been split by immigration—some remaining in the home country while others immigrated to the United States. The aging network faces the difficulty of developing the variety of programs effectively targeted at the needs and desires of all of these groups.

CHANGING COHORTS

In many locations, senior center or adult day care programs have settled into a pattern based on the background of current cohorts of older persons. At the same time, senior centers have also noted that their participants are aging in place and that they are attracting fewer numbers of younger participants than in the past. Some activities, such as trips, appear to attract younger participants, but other activities, including crafts and recreational activities, seem to have less appeal, particularly to men.

The problem of attracting new participants to a number of current programs and services will probably increase as the twenty-first century progresses. Many baby boomers born after the end of World War II have substantially more education and more financial resources than their predecessors. Their pensions and savings allow them to undertake a variety of activities, and their educational background makes them more demanding about the programs they find worthwhile. The aging network faces the challenge of developing the programs and services that will be attractive to the baby boomers and the cohorts of older people that will follow them. The success of initiatives such as ElderHostel indicates that many alternatives are available.

CHANGING HEALTH CARE

The fee-for-service health care system that served generations of Americans is rapidly disappearing. As Americans became accustomed to health insurance as a component of their employment, employers began to find health care an increasing part of their costs. It also appeared that older employees and retirees accounted for a larger percentage of health care costs. With the growth of new health technology and increased doctor and hospital fees, the traditional approach to health care began to shift dramatically in the 1980s.

Rather than hospitals being paid according to how long a patient stayed in the hospital, the new system paid fixed rates based on the patient's diagnosis. Health maintenance organizations and a variety of other arrangements have encouraged the growth of plans where physicians are on salary arrangements, or are provided a fixed amount for each patient they serve (capitation). With encouragement from the federal government, health maintenance organizations have been recruiting older persons as members.

The overall impact of these and other changes in the health care system is not yet clear. There have been complaints by some older persons about restrictions on needed health care. There have also been complaints that health maintenance organizations are only interested in recruiting healthy older people who will not utilize many services while leaving less healthy older persons to the Medicare program. The Medicare program now faces at least three very evident challenges.

The first challenge is to determine what services should be covered. For example, should medical programs to help individuals deal with obesity be covered? If the answer to this question is no, then what should be the limitations on coverage and what criteria should be used to determine these limits?

Whatever the limits placed on services, it is evident that the growing numbers of older people will mean expanded expenses for the Medicare program. The second challenge is to determine how this money should be obtained. Should general tax revenues be used or should Medicare deductibles and premiums be raised to cover the increased costs? Medicare premiums have moved up substantially in the last few years. These raises may have to continue unless new sources of funding the program are found. Although new initiatives such as coverage for prescription drugs are obviously very important for the health of older people, this benefit will be costly for Medicare. Its initial premium of approximately $32 may not be sustainable for any length of time. The aging network must be able to ensure that programs such as information, assistance, and ombudsmen help older people in their efforts to receive the health care they need. The third, and not necessarily the easiest challenge, will be to ensure that older people know what their Medicare benefits are and how to access these programs.

CHANGING PUBLIC IMAGES

In the 1960s and 1970s, requests for funding of aging programs and services received sympathetic responses in Washington and in state legislatures. During the 1980s, the responses became less positive. For the first time, older Americans were seen as well-off individuals, an "interest" group intent on preserving programs that were only of benefit to them. As the numbers of younger workers continued to decline and the number of older individuals and retirees increased, attacks on Social Security and Medicare grew. Fears about the economy and federal deficits also promoted a view that changes in these programs had to be undertaken.

For the Medicare program, this meant cutting back expenditures by reducing reimbursements to physicians or hospitals and requiring older individuals to pay higher Medicare deductibles or Part B premiums. For Social Security, this meant proposals to again raise the age of eligibility for full benefits or to privatize the program.

Funding aging programs and services also became a low priority in Congress. When the Older Americans Act reauthorization of 1992 ended in 1995, a new reauthorization was not signed into law until 2000. Part of the delay may have stemmed from disputes about particular components of the Act, particularly the older employment section. It was clear, however, that reauthorization of programs and services for older persons was less important to Congress than finding mechanisms to ensure that these efforts did not become more costly to the federal budget.

LONG-TERM SERVICES

Whatever the changes in public perception of the aged, it is evident that services for this population must be long term in nature rather than oriented to short-term crises. In a senior center, long-term services means the planning of programs for members who will attend the center for many years. The same is true of adult day care centers oriented to very frail older individuals. Even term educational programs must be offered in a framework that emphasizes continued intellectual growth rather than discrete one-time short courses.

The most pressing and the most costly initiatives in the next few decades will be for long-term care intended to assist severely impaired older persons, including patients with Alzheimer's disease. Nursing homes, home care, and adult day care are the most widely discussed elements in these efforts. Private long-term care insurance that pays for home care services and nursing homes is an important innovation, but its current high cost limits its appeal to many older persons. This need is clearly seen by providers of adult day care programs who are concerned about becoming eligible for Medicare reimbursement, particularly as the population targeted for this service changes:

> We certainly need more adult day programs. . . . We all know of areas in our communities that have no program, or are underserved. But, be aware. The field has changed, and continues to change. Fifteen years ago, the population we were serving was not as medically needy. Today the folks we serve are much more physically frail. [Schull, 1997, p. 3]

Day care programs must meet the challenges of a changing clientele. New types of long-term efforts, particularly assisted living, are also finding that their residents require extensive services. Some facilities are unprepared or uninterested in providing services for frailer residents, including services for residents suffering from dementia. As a recent investigative report indicates, oversight and standards for assisted living remain deficient. In both Massachusetts and Oregon, assisted living facilities are inspected every second year. In California, they are inspected every five years (Assisted living, 2005). The current challenges for this and other forms of residential programs for older people include better definition of the parameters of their programs and the development and enforcement of standards that ensure adequate living standards for residents.

INNOVATION AND THE AGING NETWORK

The role of the public aging network in long-term care and in the provision of programs and services to older people is more in question now than it has ever been since the passage of the Older Americans Act in 1965. As Hudson and Kingson (1991) reaffirm, there can be no question that the intent of the Older Americans Act was to serve all older persons, regardless of their situation. Over time, as the economic situation of the older population has improved, it has seemed more important to stress the needs of economically needy, socially needy, and impaired older persons.

To some extent, the growth of provisions in the OAA is a positive reflection of the growth of the field of aging and groups concerned about specific issues. It is questionable, however, whether one major piece of legislation based on the administrative structure of State Units on Aging and Area Agencies on Aging can effectively embody all of these concerns. There are arguments that AAAs should become coordinators of all community programs and services. In the American social welfare structure, coordination is a difficult task because of the myriad administrative arrangements that exist to provide services at state and local levels. Many of the most crucial programs and services for the aged are not under the control of the Administration on Aging. These include transportation, housing, education, and health care. Because the American social welfare structure is organized along these functional lines (e.g., transportation, an agency concerned with a specific population group (e.g., the aged) has difficulty pulling together the resources and overcoming the "turf" issues that will enable it to mount effective methods. In the 1960s, the federal Office of Economic Opportunity, organized to coordinate programs for the poor, encountered the same obstacles. Even if it were possible to implement, coordination of programs and services for older people by the AAA would not necessarily reduce costs for long-term care, delay nursing home placement, or lead to positive changes in functioning among older people (Fortinsky, 1991).

The expansion of the field of aging has also brought many new groups into the service provision arena. Hospitals, concerned about reduced numbers of inpatients, are promoting outpatient and in-home services. Private firms have begun to develop products specifically geared to older people, and the housing industry has become extensively involved in the potential retirement and life-care community markets. Voluntary agencies now provide services similar to those offered through public agencies. Employers are beginning to offer elder care programs for employees. Private case managers have developed a network around the country to serve families who can afford these services; private adult day care programs have also begun to appear in some locales. The public sector, which involves State Units on Aging and Area Agencies on Aging, is now only one element in an enlarged service delivery complex concerned about older people (Quirk, 1991). The failure of federal funding to grow has made it difficult for AoA to maintain its past programs at an adequate level.

One possible source of revenue is cost-sharing. The question of whether sharing the costs of the programs with consumers is the appropriate mechanism for financing efforts of AAAs and State Units on Aging is a major point for debate. A second method of increasing income is for public agencies to offer services to corporations. Many Area Agencies on Aging are currently involved in the development of elder care services in the workplace. These services include education, caregiver consultation, and case management.

Cost-sharing will not resolve the issue of future directions for the public aging network and, in particular, the role of the Older Americans Act. Alternatives to the approach currently embodied in the latest amendments of the Older Americans Act are possible. This approach would narrow the Act's focus to a few priority services that are targeted at frail and impaired older persons and low-income elderly. Although this approach would clarify the intent of the Act, it would certainly negate its universal emphasis and, over time, perhaps result in means-testing for eligibility.

A change in direction cannot be made without extensive discussion and evaluation of the effectiveness of programs operated through the aging network. Unfortunately, evaluation of these programs is weak, partly due to a lack of standards. Rather than the effects of a program on any number of criteria, reports by AAAs, the state, and the AoA stress numbers of participants, numbers of meals served, or numbers of older workers placed in jobs. Kutza (1991) views these "failures to be self-critical" (p. 67) as weakening the aging network. The reluctance to be self-critical, however, also reflects the maturity of the aging network, and the self-protective desire of agencies to ensure their continued funding and existence. Full-scale valid evaluations of aging network programs now confront an aging network less concerned about innovation than survival, particularly in a period of economic uncertainty. The dilemma of increased demands, but limited resources, may force an intensive reexamination of the effectiveness of programs, the simplification of access to important programs and services, and the development of programs designed to deal with some of the most difficult remaining problems, such as long-term care.

These goals cannot be accomplished in a framework that views programs and services for the aged as separate from those for other populations. Social welfare advocates must unite in a framework that sees the needs of children, the aged, minority populations, and other groups as interrelated rather than competitive. A failure to bridge seeming differences in needs will mean continued competition for social welfare dollars—a competition that will eventually defeat the best intents of all advocacy groups.

REFERENCES

Assisted living. (2005). *Consumer Reports, 70*(7), 28–33.

Fortinsky, R. (1991). Coordinated, comprehensive community care and the Older Americans Act. *Generations, 15,* 39–42.

Hudson, R., & Kingson, E. (1991). Inclusive and fair: The case for universality in social programs. *Generations, 15,* 51–56.

Kutza, E. (1991). The Older Americans Act of 2000: What should it be? *Generations, 15,* 65–68.

National Center for Health Statistics. (2003). *Health, United States, 2003: Life expectancy at birth, at 65 years of age and 75 years of age, according to race and sex: United States, selected years 1900–2001.* Retrieved February 10, 2005, from http://www.cdc.gov/nchs/data/hus/tables/2003/03hus027.pdf

Quirk, D. (1991). The aging network: An agenda for the nineties and beyond. *Generations, 15,* 23–26.

Schull, P. (1997) Adult day services: Future directions: From a national perspective. *Respite Report, Special Issue: Adult Day Services: 10 Years in 2 Days, Summer.* Wake Forest, NC: Bowman Gray School of Medicine.

APPENDIX

National Nonprofit Resources Groups in Aging

Administration on Aging (AoA), Office of Human Development, U.S. Department of Health and Human Services, Washington, DC, 20402; (202) 245-0213. http://www.aoa.gov

Coordinates programs, services, and research to help older Americans. Administers and authorizes funds for major programs. Operates National Clearinghouse on Aging, which collects, stores, and disseminates information about the elderly. Responds to all inquiries from the general public. State agencies and local Area Agencies on Aging offer consultation, grant application assistance, program information, and help to individuals.

AoA is the major starting point for all program information. As advocate for the elderly, AoA is committed to coordinated action of all federal agencies with programs and services involving older people and to the development of comprehensive information and referral programs. If you cannot locate your area agency in the phone directory, contact the mayor or local executive's office.

Publications: *Aging*, monthly magazine updating national, state, and local resources, legislation, and agency news.

Other: *AoA Fact Sheets*, technical assistance documents, and other materials to meet the needs of the aged, general public, planners, and gerontologists. Publication list available.

Food & Nutrition Service (FNS), U.S. Department of Agriculture, Washington, DC, 20036; (703) 305-2262. http://www.fns.usda.gov/fns

Coordinates federal food stamp programs. Information available here or more directly from food stamp offices in most major cities. Offices may provide consultation or speakers in areas of nutrition or food

243

management. Surplus food for use by nonprofit, tax-exempt, residental institutions may be available from FNS; contact FNS offices.

Editor's note: Although food distribution for congregate dining programs may be coordinated by this office, the Nutrition Program for the Elderly is directed by AoA, and inquiries should be addressed to AoA or its area agencies. Meals delivered to homebound elderly as part of this program may be paid for with food stamps; contact food stamp offices for information.

AARP (formerly American Association of Retired Persons), 601 E Street, NW, Washington, DC, 20049; (888) 682-2277. http://www.aarp.gov

National organization of older Americans with 2,000 local chapters. Services include legislative representation at the federal and state levels, mail-order pharmacy service for prescription medicine, supplemental "Medigap" policies, and a variety of programs ranging from retirement education to bereavement counseling and tax preparation assistance.

Publications: *Modern Maturity,* bimonthly magazine of general interest and information for retired people; *AARP Bulletin,* and a variety of other publications.

American Society on Aging, 833 Market Street, Suite 511, San Francisco, CA, 94103; (800) 537-9728. http://www.asaging.org

The ASA provides a national forum for the discussion of major programmatic and policy issues in aging for practitioners and academics. Society based projects (e.g., Aging in the Neighborhood), conferences, and publications are supported by a national membership.

Publications: *Aging Today, Generations* (quarterly journal), *ASA Connections.*

Asociacion Nacional Por Personas Mayores (National Association for Spanish Speaking Elderly), 234 East Colorado Boulevard, Suite 300, Pasadena, CA, 91101; (626) 564-1988. http://www.anppm.org.

This organization was founded to inform policy makers and the general public regarding the status and needs of elderly Hispanics and other low-income elderly persons. The Asociacion advocates for the needs of elderly Hispanics, and conducts research as well as conferences on the needs and status of older Hispanics.

Gerontological Society, 1035 15th Street, NW, Suite 250, Washington, DC, 20005; (202) 842-1275. http://www.geron.org

Promotes scientific study of aging and application of research findings. Four areas of education stressed at annual meeting: biology, clinical medicine, behavioral and social sciences, social planning, research, and practice.

Publications: *Journals of Gerontology,* bimonthly journal of original scientific research (emphasis on data analysis, methodology); *Gerontologist,* bimonthly journal of applied research (interpretive).

Gray Panthers, 733 15th Street, NW, Suite 437, Washington, DC, 20005; (800) 280-5362. http://www.graypanthers.org

Eschews special interest focus; advocates change that will benefit people of all ages. Nationally, monitors issues of social justice and joins coalition groups speaking out on issues of health care, consumer fraud, nursing home reform, and public transportation.

National Asian Pacific Center on Aging, 1511 Third Avenue, Suite 914, Seattle, WA, 98101; (206) 624-1221. http://www.napca.org

An advocacy organization, the NAPCA develops demonstration programs and ongoing direct service programs. NAPCA also identifies community-based resources for the Asian/Pacific Island elderly and disseminates information throughout the nation via resources directories and a fax-on-demand system.

National Association of Area Agencies on Aging, 1730 Rhode Island Avenue, NW, Suite 1200, Washington, DC, 20036; (202) 872-0888. http://www.n4a.org

An organization that represents the Area Agencies on Aging around the U.S.

National Association of State Units on Aging, 1201 15th Street, NW, Suite 350, Washington, DC, 20005; (202) 898-2578. http://www.nasua.org

An organization that represents the state offices on aging around the country.

National Caucus and Center on the Black Aged, 1220 L Street, NW, Suite 800, Washington, DC, 20005; (202) 637-8400. http://ncba-aged.org

Advocates attention and programs for the Black aged. Recommends public policies responsive to the needs of the older Black American. Conducts research, curriculum development in the area of Black aging, training of Black professionals in gerontology, training of Black elderly to assume leadership roles in services to Black aged, and aids in participation of minority social organizations and businesses in service delivery to the elderly. Also conducts employment program for rural Black elderly and operates elderly housing. National and local conferences on black aged.

Publications: Newsletters, job bank publications; reports on health, research, curriculum, and theoretical and policy perspectives on Black aged.

National Council on the Aging (NCOA), 300 D Street, SW, Suite 801, Washington, DC, 20024; (202) 479-1200. http://www.ncoa.org

Professionally oriented organization that represents a variety of service providers working in the field of aging. Members include senior centers, adult day service centers, area agencies on aging, faith congregations, senior housing facilities, employment services, and other consumer organizations. NCOA monitors legislation and conducts research and special projects through constituent units such as the National Institute of Senior Centers, the National Institute of Senior Housing, and the National Institute on Community-Based Long-Term Care.

National Hispanic Council on Aging, 1341 Connecticut Avenue, NW, 4th floor, Washington, DC, 20036; (202) 429-0789. http://nhcoa.org

Established in 1979, NHCOA has chapters throughout the United States. Through its publications and demonstration projects, NHCOA keeps its members informed about important issues facing Latino seniors in many important areas of life including education, health, housing, and community development.

National Indian Council on Aging, 10501 Montgomery Boulevard, NE, Albuquerque, NM, 87111; (505) 292-2001. http://www.nicoa.org

Formed by tribal chairs in 1976, the overall purpose of the council is to bring about improved comprehensive services to the Indian and Alaskan Native elderly. The council encourages legislative action, communication, and cooperation with service provider agencies, dissemination of information to the Indian communities, and supportive resources, and, when necessary, intercedes with appropriate agencies to provide access to resources.

Index

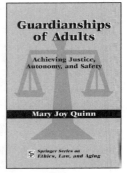

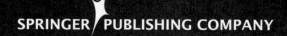
SPRINGER / PUBLISHING COMPANY

End-of-Life Stories
Crossing Disciplinary Boundaries

Donald E. Gelfand, PhD, Richard Raspa, PhD
Sherylyn H. Briller, PhD
Stephanie Myers Schim, PhD, RN, APRN, CNAA, BC, Editors

This book provides a variety of narratives about end-of-life experiences contributed by members of the Wayne State University End-of-Life Interdisciplinary Project. Each of the narratives is then analyzed from three different disciplinary perspectives. These analyses broaden how specific end-of-life narratives can be viewed from different dimensions and help students, researchers, and practitioners see the important and varied meanings that end-of-life experiences have at the level of the individual, the family, and the community. In addition, the narratives include end-of-life experiences of individuals from a variety of ethnic and racial backgrounds.

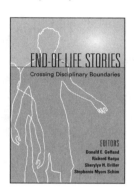

Partial Contents:

2005   218pp   0-8261-2675-8   hardcover

11 West 42nd Street, New York, NY 10036-8002 • Fax: 212-941-7842
Order Toll-Free: 877-687-7476 • Order On-line: www.springerpub.com